Ousting

Sniffles

How to build iron-strong immune system

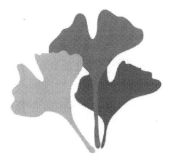

Dr. Dorothy Adamiak, ND

LiveUthing Press

ISBN-13: 978-1981850570
ISBN-10: 1981850570

Disclaimer

All information provided in this book is for educational purposes only. The information is not intended as a substitute for the medical advice of physicians. The reader should regularly consult a physician in matters relating to his/her health and particularly with respect to any symptoms that may require diagnosis or medical attention. This information is not intended to replace clinical judgment or guide individual patient care in any manner.

Use of this book implies your acceptance of this disclaimer.

Table of Contents

Preface

Nothing is random in health, definitely not the works of the immune system. Sniffles aren't random either, even though they may seem so. There is a reason why the bugs have a fondness for you, not anyone else. Have you ever seen a gang of giraffes packing up in Africa and heading towards the snow-covered continents? I bet you haven't! Giraffes hate cold. They lounge in warm climates, where they find food and comfort. Germs are not any different. They cozy themselves in favorable environment and preferably in a host with weak defenses. They won't be sticking around hostile noses and wicked white blood cells.

Rest assured, your whiffer does not need any snake oils, yearly memberships, or secret ingredients, but solid defenses, strong membranes, and germ-proofed interior. Perfect health does not need a pile of pills or a life-long friendship with a pharmacist, but a few intelligent lifestyle changes. So read, discover, and transition to an iron-strong immune system.

Now, off to the first chapter, I mean to your best health yet.... because a red nose glows well on Rudolf, not you.

DrD

Health Tools

"Ousting Sniffles" is full of practical suggestions. Occasionally you may want to look up a product, test, or additional information mentioned in the book. Whatever you are looking for you will be able to find on two of our websites:

DrDNaturopath.com

LiveUthing.com

These website tell our life story and share clinical pearls that I have gathered over 20 years practicing as a naturopathic physician. They have hundreds of articles on health, quizzes, and links to health tools you may never thought existed.

Chapter 1

Is it a cold or is it a flu?

Which one is it then: a cold or a flu? Although English language is decisively clear, the symptoms may not be. The truth is that when the initial chill takes over the body it is really hard to tell. But as the malady plows ahead the differences get easier to spot. It is true that both, common cold and flu are due to a virus and can start with a runny nose, but with a little bit of an insight, they can be fully distinguished. Their symptoms, severity, timing, and also prognosis are quite different.

A primer on common cold

Did you know that common cold is the most frequent infectious disease in humans? That means "kinda" everyone gets it. An average adult will get two to four common colds a year and those will likely appear during winter. Thus if you are statistically plagued by two colds a winter, you fit perfectly in our two-sniffles-a-year society, but if your nose acts up every month, that's something to look at.

The cold season runs between September and April. Interestingly, chilling weather is not the only factor blamed for it. The resurgence and spread of the virus during that time is also blamed on schools. Kids are said to be a major contributor to the spread of the illness. I bet you have witnessed a mucoid bubble coming out of a six-year old nose, haven't you?

The absence of a droopy snort can be deceiving. Six-year-olds are not the only ones passing on the germs. Many adults also transmit common cold viruses, but without the obvious nasal gunk. Half of common colds cases are so mild that they can barely be noticed. The other, less fortunate half, may not be able to hide it that easy. The most unfortunate may even end up with a combo that resembles a case of mild flu, a combination of sore throat, cough, headache, fatigue, and muscle soreness however, without the fever.

Typically cold sniffles last one to two weeks. Residual cough may linger up to eighteen days. Common cold seldom amounts to more than a few nuisance symptoms, but in a small fraction of immuno-compromised individuals it may lead to pneumonia.[1] Despite being mild on the body, common cold is not mild on the US economy. It accounts for 40% of all time lost from work and total economic impact due to common cold exceeds $20 billion per year.

Common cold virus is said to infect upper respiratory tract. It lives in a nose, sinuses, throat, and voice box, but those don't act up with symptoms the minute the virus lands there, only about sixteen hours afterwards. Can you get the virus if you haven't met anybody that was cold-stricken? Sure! The cold virus can be sneaky. It either floats quietly in the air or waits patiently on contaminated objects. Since we cannot stop breathing and our hands constantly touch computer keyboards, door knobs, and banknotes prevention is not so easy.

Resist the urge to spray anti-microbial mist into the air or clean-scrub your furniture till the surface gets raw. Sterilizing the environment to avoid the viruses is not only highly unpractical, but also counterproductive. People that live in sterile conditions end up with a dysfunctional immune system, which means they get more prone to being a microbial host.

Currently we don't know of any medications or herbal remedies that would *guarantee* to shorten the duration of the cold. For now, the best way to treat it is to never get it. Don't even think about antibiotics. They won't help. Antibiotics are designed to kill bacteria, not viruses.

Treating common cold with antibiotics does nothing for the symptoms. Instead it weakens the immune system and supports the development of antibiotic-resistant bacteria. Too bad, because due to patient pressure one third of all common cold infections end up with a prescription for antibiotics.

Patients like pills. Pills can do miracles. That`s why even a mild sickness like common cold drives ill-stricken to pharmacies and health food stores in droves. Did you know that Americans spend $2.9 billion on over-the-counter drugs and another $400 million on prescription medicines for cold symptom relief each year?

A word about flu

Similarly to common cold, flu can be caused by several different viruses, which belong to a few distinctive types and families. These vary in infectiveness and severity.

A flu virus from family named "A" is the real trouble maker. It can cause severe illness. "A" has been responsible for several flu pandemics, which included Bird flu in 2004 and Swine flu in 2009. Viruses from family "B" are less common than family "A" and so far have not been responsible for any massive outbreaks. They also only infect humans, thus transmission via animals is unlikely. Viruses from family "C", which can infect animals, are even less common than "B". These are responsible only for minor illness in children.

Flu strikes in winter, peaking when the temperatures dip the lowest. February sees the majority of cases, although officially the flu season runs from December to March. During its peak month, flu infects about 0.3% of the population, or 3 people in 1,000.[2] Although that does not seem like much, flu can cause an economic havoc. Flu costs the United States approximately 10 billion dollars a year. Pandemic can increase this number to hundreds of billions of dollars.

Flu starts with sudden onset, high fever, extreme fatigue and severe body aches. The symptoms may be so severe that they can completely disable a person. This seldom happens with a common cold, which presents less of a challenge to the immune system.

Influenza spreads through airborne droplets, infected objects, and direct contact with the infected. But not everyone who is in contact with the virus will automatically get the flu. Only 67% will develop any symptoms. The remaining 33% will not even sneeze once or be aware of contact with the germ. For those life continues as usual, as if nothing happened.[3]

You may wonder what makes these people more fortunate than the other two thirds. May it be luck, genetics, or the vitamin C they just swallowed? I believe none of that. This apparent luck is simply a manifestation of a stronger immune system. Solid body defences are not random, genetic, or incidental, but they result from a combination of body biochemistry and the environment, both of which I will explain in the upcoming chapters.

Flu vs cold comparison chart

Symptom	Cold	Flu
Onset	Slow, in days	Sudden, in hours
Fever	None or low	Yes, high
Headache	None or mild	Yes, severe
Stuffy nose	Yes	Frequent
Dry cough	Yes	Frequent
Muscle pain	None or mild	Yes
Fatigue	None or mild	Yes
Duration	7-10 days	3-7 days

Chapter 2

Don't kill the fever!

I have to say my mom was a very wise woman. When I was growing up I was plagued with fevers, but she knew exactly what to do about them. She did not panic. To her a fever was not a sickness, but the necessary response to it. She did not give me any pills to suppress the heat unless the temperature got dangerously high. She knew better. Without the fever my body defenses would stifle and leave me with lower chances for recovery.

Today's parents are very different. Americans spent over two billion dollars on antipyretics and analgesics in 2015 alone.[4]

There are two reasons for such a shift. The first one is that we now have different priorities. We are too busy for lying around. We don't have time for health nuisances, aches, pains, inflammation and fevers. We have other plans. We want to go shopping, visit friends, or simply be productive. Life outside the bed is much more rewarding. Staying under covers to swelter is far from fun.

The second reason is that we confuse fevers with infections and symptoms with diseases. We believe that lack of fever means lack of sickness. We think that once the fever is gone, so is the virus. We also believe that lack of discomfort equals a healthy body. As a result our efforts are focused on erasing the symptoms, rather than boosting body powers.

It is baffling, but our entire medical system has been taken over by this ideology. Notice that doctors' efforts are focused on killing pathogens, reducing discomfort and fighting inflammation, not on restoring balance to the immune system or helping it work better. The bias to treat the end effects (mucus, fever, cough) rather than the causes (weak immune system) is rampant and plain wrong.

Fever is not the sickness you are after

Let me illustrate. You are chopping vegetables in the kitchen. The phone rings. You look up to see who`s calling and in the moment of inattention you nick your finger. Not a big deal, yet it is obvious that your skin is pierced. You dab the finger with a tissue and look at it intently to assess the damage. The cut isn't much to talk about. No stitches needed and a band aid will do.

A small cut won't occupy your mind for too long. It always heals. And even though the nature will do its thing without you noticing, I would like you to know how it actually happens. Notice the predictable sequence: first you cut your finger, which only then gets red, swollen, hot and painful. Let me stress it again: first injury, then inflammation. Never the other way around. Cooling inflammation doesn`t prevent injury. Putting ice on the finger before the phone call can`t blunt the knife or make you less clumsy.

The resulting red finger is not there for fashion. There is a reason why nature blesses you with a painfully engorged stub after the cut. It is not to punish you for clumsiness, but to ensure a quick recuperation of your precious appendage. In the attempt to do that the blood rushes to the injured site and brings an army of battle-hungry immune cells. These are ready to fight off any pathogens that may be trying to sneak inside the finger through the breached skin.

Red blood cells follow. They flock in to the site armed with oxygen that will be used as ammunition against the germs. As both cells work in synchrony and regenerative processes ensues, expect an uneventful recovery. In a few days your finger will be just like new.

Let's stop here and ponder for a minute. What do you think would happen if you interfere with the healing process? What would happen if you stop the rush of blood and the oxygen to the finger? On the one side, you will not have to deal with a puffy extremity, but on the other side your pinky may succumb to a tragic fate. Nasty bacteria do not sleep and a finger void of defenses is an easy target. Considering the consequences, would you take a comfort pill that voids the pinky of heat and bulge or rather stick the fight out? I'd rather have a healing stiffer for a few days than an open wound for the unforeseeable future. Rest assured, when allowed, things go back to normal. When the intruders are taken care of heat and pain simply disappear. No fight, no battlefield.

Fever is a friend

Inflammations and fevers are not random and although people think of them as enemies, they are their best friends. It is the germs you are after, not the fever. Don't suppress the fever, because everyone else does so. Remove the underlying cause, not your body defenses.

Studies show that fever lowering practices actually prolong many illnesses. Fever reduction leads to slower recovery in viral illnesses including flu.[5] The use of aspirin and acetaminophen during the sickness makes head congestion worse and contributes to longer viral shedding.[6] In the United States fever suppression causes at least extra 700 deaths per year from influenza alone.

Fever fights cancer

Fever is an amazing defense and its power goes beyond killing viruses. Fever can elevate the immune system to such a high degree that it can bring about a spontaneous tumor remission. First it was just a rumor saying that tumors disappear after a high fever, but systemic observations and formal studies confirmed that a period of high fever can in fact initiate a regression of cancerous lumps. Not long after the power of fever was proven, heat therapy became a popular form of cancer treatment. Did you know that normal cells and cancer cells have different temperature sensitivity? While normal cells survive temperature of 42-43°C, cancerous ones do not. High fever is lethal to cancer cells as they die above 42°C. Meanwhile, the ordinary body cells can handle temperatures of up to 47°C.

Fever therapy is not our most modern invention. It has been used with success since the mid of 19th century and it was first used to treat ovarian and breast cancers.[7] Today fever therapy evolved to a highly sophisticated high-tech treatment for tumors. The therapy has been adopted by modern clinics under the name of hyperthermia, where either local or full body heat is applied. Heat treatment is now used with success in variety of cancers including sarcoma, melanoma, cancers of the head and neck, brain, lung, esophagus, breast, bladder, rectum, liver, appendix, cervix, and peritoneal lining (mesothelioma).[8]

Hyperthermia is a non-toxic, natural, and very effective way to boost the immune system. This simulated fever unleashes full immune body fighting potential. Higher temperatures increase replication of the immune cells, which in turn boosts the number of active fighters. And since fever increases the metabolic rate and speeds up the blood flow, these cells can reach any remote tissue in practically no time.

Fever is a great health-keeper. Fever is an ultimate demonstration of the immune system prowess, its strength and potential, and not an unnecessary nuisance that takes productive days away. An occasional fever should be welcomed and never suppressed.

And just as heat boosts the body defenses, lack of it may signal immune system weakness. Did you know that cancer patients frequently report being fever-free for many years prior to the diagnosis and that there is a significant correlation between history of infectious diseases and cancer risk? It is simple as that: people who don`t suffer from infections have an increased cancer risk.

The risk of malignancy goes up for people who never had mumps, measles, or rubella. It also goes up for people who do not have the usual flus and colds. The highest risk for cancers is seen in people with the lowest incidence of infections, or the lowest infection index.

Large scale studies managed to establish how specific infections affect cancer odds. Below is a simplified version of the correlation. 1.0 means that there is a normal (non-increased) risk for cancer. Higher number indicates increased odds for cancer diagnosis.

- 1.0 - with history of fevers
- 2.6 - for missing history of infectious organ diseases
- 5.7 - for missing history of common colds,
- 15.1 - for missing history of fever [9]

The numbers are so shocking that they should make us reconsider the value of fever-producing infections. Nowadays where everyone is potentially threatened by a cancer epidemic, an occasional fever may turn out to be the greatest prevention method nature has to offer.

You get the picture. People who get no fevers aren't necessarily the healthiest among us. They may actually be the ones that are getting the raw end of the immune bargain. With a whooping 15.1 risk increase for cancer, there is not much to boast about.

What does a doctor do when she gets a fever?

I don't know what other health care practitioners are doing, but I can share with you my own routine for sickly days. You may be wondering, whether I do what most people do: swallow a highly potent fever killer, go to work, and carry on as usual. I don't!

To me nature says: stop, we need to rearrange things in your body! I listen. I shut down my schedule, take out cozy pyjamas, fluff my bed, and keep three warm blankets handy. I line up filtered water, herbal teas, vitamin C, and some homeopathic concoctions on the counter. I may use them later.

Then I close the door, open the window, sneak under the covers, and stay until baking time. I know it will feel hot and uncomfortable until I break a sweat and my body cools down. I want my sweat to be so profuse that it runs rivers down my body. I know that hot-cold cycles may continue for a while, and although the process is uncomfortable, I see it as a necessity, not an option. If it gets too cold I drink a hot tea or pile more blankets on myself to get the fire going. If it gets too hot I stick a leg out just to get a partial relief while waiting for sweat to reappear. My aim is to work with nature, not against it.

It is true, fever time can be miserable. It can change personalities and turn otherwise pleasant people into needy, irritable whiners that groan, bitch, and complain. But regardless how bad the transformation may appear, this short-lived family disruption may be totally worth it. Fever not only leaves the viruses behind, but also dissolves those ugly cancer cells. Don`t kid yourself. No amount of detoxifying juices, enemas, and purges can do what that one flu can do for health. It may sound weird, but I like my flu because of this.

Caveat: if your body is unable to mount a fever, your white blood cells are decimated, or you are on medication that suppresses natural immune responses, you won't benefit from a short-lived infection. Only robust bodies capable of putting up a strong fight can succeed in battling viruses. If you are not sure where you stand and what your immune system is doing, don't play the hero. Seek a professional that can guide you back to health.

Chapter 3

Light up your fire

What if you keep on having infection after infection or are constantly on the verge of "getting something?" Should you fluff up your bed and line up herbal teas for three months in a row? No need! There is a better way.

It is very easy to blame a tenacious virus for sniffling misfortunes, but the truth is that chronic infections hunt either those who keep on suppressing their fevers or those who "naturally" have low body temperature.

Viruses love cold bodies. That's why flus and colds find victims in winter. For example, rhinovirus, the most common cold virus replicates preferentially at 32°C (89.6°F). If it can't find its super-comfy low-temp spot it will settle in a tissue that is between 33°C (91.4°F) and 35°C (95.0°F). Since rhinovirus does not like heat, the most effective way to end its presence is to keep the body warm.

Did you know that core body temperature is one of the most important factors in setting the pace for the immune system? A mere 1°C (1.8°F) drop in body temperature causes 40% decline in the immune function![10] Now think about it. If an optimal body temperature is 36.6°C (97.9°F), but your body works at 35°C (95°F), where do you think your immune system weakness comes from?

Core temperature sets the pace for more than just the immune system. It orchestrates the entire body. Lower temperature can shut down many organ functions, deactivate vital metabolic enzymes, change hormone production, and alter neurotransmitter transmission. Lack of body heat can stop cellular communication and make symptoms and diseases appear.

Below-optimal body temperature is extremely common and so are problems associated with it. Here is a partial list of those: recurrent colds and sub-clinical viral infections, fatigue, headaches, migraines, PMS, easy weight gain, depression, irritability, fluid retention, anxiety and panic attacks, hair loss, poor memory, poor concentration, low sex drive, unhealthy nails, dry skin and hair, cold intolerance, heat intolerance, low motivation, low ambition, insomnia, allergies, acne, carpal tunnel syndrome, asthma, odd swallowing sensations, constipation, irritable bowel syndrome, muscle and joint aches, slow healing, sweating abnormalities, Raynaud's Phenomenon, itchiness, irregular periods, easy bruising, ringing of the ears, flushing, bad breath, dry eyes/ blurred vision.[11]

Many of us try to fix the above ailments with lotions, potions, teas and pills without having any inclination to check body temperature. In too many cases instead of success, frustration follows. The ailments recur with vengeance, because low body temperature prevents healing response even after application of the most-indicated therapies. The biochemical pathways needed for the repair are simply either too slow or completely shut down. The moral of the story is: know your body temperature before trying to dry up your sniffles. You can spare yourself a major disappointment.

Testing for core body temperature

First, arm yourself with a reliable thermometer. Since your immune system assessment depends on its accuracy, don't try to settle for any old clunker. Also pick three to seven consecutive days to perform the test. Schedule them while you are not acutely sick, in chills or spiking fever. If you are a menstruating woman, account for two different temperature phases that occur during the menstrual cycle. The body is naturally cooler in the first two weeks of a 28-day rhythm. The other two weeks are likely to show a spike on a thermometer. To see your most immunologically vulnerable point perform the test when temperature is at its lowest, which is right after the menstruation.

Do the test in the morning before you start your day. This way you will avoid misleading temperature spikes from physical activity. The best time for the test is right after waking, when your body is still cozying in bed under warm covers. When done properly, the test will reflect your resting metabolic rate.

Body temperature is an important health marker. It not only can tell how fast the body burns fat, but also whether the glands such as thyroid or adrenals are doing well. Lack of proper thermoregulation can shut down circulation, detoxification, and the immune system. The ideal basal body temperature (BBT) is 36.6°C (97.8°F). Acceptable BBT is between 36.0°C (96.8°F) and 37.0°C (98.6°F). If your body temperature is consistently outside this range, you will need to investigate the causes.

Use the chart below to record your findings.

Day	Temperature
Day 1	
Day 2	
Day 3	
Day 4	
Day 5	
Day 6	
Day 7	

There are three very common conditions that are known to down-regulate the temperature. These are: low adrenals, low thyroid, and diabetes/pre-diabetes. My clinical experience taught me that nearly every single patient with low BBT has either one of these conditions. When it comes to detection of the reasons behind low BBT you are on your own. Few doctors would be interested in low BBT unless they are reviving a hypothermia patient.

A primer to rule out underlying conditions

Your journey to better BBT does not start with waiting for your doctor to tell you what to do, but to actively engage in self-discovery. That`s not very difficult. Low adrenals, low thyroid, or blood sugar swings can be easily tested. It would be helpful if your doctor is on your side, but in case he has no interest in the suggested tests, you can order those online.

1) **Adrenals:** Absolutely the best test for the adrenal function is a 4-point saliva cortisol. You can purchase a kit online, collect your sample and send it back to the lab for analysis. Adrenal assessment is based on diurnal cortisol pattern. Cortisol, a stress hormone peaks in the morning and is followed by steady decline of the hormone for the rest of the day. Cortisol pattern reflect adrenal function and can detect their over- or under-activity. Underactive adrenals are very common in chronically stressed or overworked individuals. They are also the most frequent underlying reason behind low BBT. If this is your case, you would need to first restore adrenal function before expecting a boost in immunity.

2) **Thyroid:** Thyroid function is best tested through a blood sample. The most basic test is called thyroid stimulating hormone (TSH) and this is also the most commonly used screen for over- and under functioning thyroid. TSH can either be bought on line or ordered though a doctor. While interpreting the results however, don't follow the ranges dictated by the lab.

They are too wide to detect minor issues, such as slow metabolism which you are after. The ranges are set only to flag a major problem, in this case a thyroid disease. Because your doctor is likely to follow the ranges, he will only alarm you when your numbers fall outside. Because you are interested in the numbers that are close, but not necessarily outside the borders, you need to see and judge the numbers yourself. Thyroid sluggishness usually follows lethargic adrenal, thus if you have both start with the latter.

3) **Blood sugar:** There are two very useful tests for screening blood sugar: HbA1C and fasting blood sugar. HbA1C averages blood glucose fluctuations in the preceding three months, while fasting blood sugar reflects one particular morning. These two tests can give you a good idea how your body handles glucose. You are not looking to diagnose yourself with diabetes, but to see whether blood sugar fluctuates sufficiently to have a negative effect on your body. Check whether your fasting glucose numbers or HbA1C either are close to the normal lab ranges or already have crossed the border. Blood sugar fluctuation whether high or low is detrimental to the immune system. High numbers fuel chronic inflammation. Low numbers drag down the defenses.

If you discover that your BBT is affected by adrenals, thyroid or fluctuating blood sugar, you will need to address them first. These may be hidden reasons for persistent sniffles. Without their correction expect the immune system to keep on falling behind.

Summary of tests:

Test	Action	Did that!
Basal Body Temperature	Do 7-day test	
Adrenal screen	Order 4-point diurnal cortisol test	
Thyroid screen	Order TSH test	
(Pre)diabetes/hypoglycemia	Order HbA1C + fasting blood sugar test	

Chapter 4

Warm up your days

How you live can strongly influence the body temperature. If you constantly feel chilled out, instead of reaching for blankets, thermogenic pills, or hot cider, consider where you live and what you eat. There may be something in your environment or your diet has a profound body cooling effect. Look for a tiny breeze under the door, partially malfunctioning heater, constantly running air conditioner, drafty working conditions, basement wetness, or habitual underdressing. Your lifestyle may be exceptionally cooling.

Check your diet as well. Cold food, frozen food, and raw food cool the body. Be smart about energetics. Leave refrigerated salads, ice creams and popsicles for hot summer days. Don`t use them during winter. If your body feels chilled avoid eating anything that is cold to touch regardless how "healthy" it may be. Frozen blueberries may not be your best choice during a cold.

There is one twist to food energetics. According to traditional Chinese and Ayurveda systems all foods carry their own thermal signature regardless whether they have been refrigerated or charcoaled. This knowledge has been an integral part of these ancient healing systems, where cooling foods have been prescribed for hot conditions and warming foods for cold ailments. For example, cinnamon which has warming properties would be given for chills, but no reputable doctor would prescribe a banana for that condition. That would be a malpractice. Banana is cooling and can drive the body into a deeper freeze.

Today, an overwhelming majority of health practitioners do not consider food thermal effect. The topic of food energetics has been completely excluded from modern medical textbooks. The result is a plethora of poor dietary recommendations. Blueberry yogurts and bananas are endorsed as health-promoting regardless of the body temperature. Be wiser. Stick to lamb, wine and cinnamon if you are chill-prone.

The full list of hot and cold foods is too long to list. Below is the shortened version so that you can get a taste of it.

Cold foods: avoid them if your BBT is low. In case these are your absolute favorites, heat them up before eating.

- Asparagus
- Bamboo shoots
- Tomato
- Water chestnut
- Banana
- Grapefruit

- Lemon
- Mango
- Melon
- Clam
- Crab
- Yoghurt

Warm foods: stick to those on a daily basis. For better effect eat them cooked, when still warm.

- Leek
- Onion
- Pepper
- Sweet potato
- Chicken
- Lamb
- Turkey
- Oats
- Quinoa
- Coffee
- Butter
- Coconut
- Trout

Besides taking a few tests, rearranging the environment and investing in warming foods, there are a few other fire boosting methods that should be on your radar. Among the most noticeable ones that bring warmth to the body are relaxing sun bathing, vigorous physical activity, and modern infrareds.

Make friends with the Sun

Sun bathing has been promoted as a favorite pastime for vacationing families, not so much as an immune-boosting therapy. Tourist agencies ensure that sun bathing means leisure time, not an unconventional virus eradicating treatment. I bet no airline company aims to fill up their planes with mucus snorting customers. Besides, emerald seas, warm sand and kids building castles create much more alluring ads than red noses and tissue piles.

We take sunny vacation, because it is fun, not because it is healthy. Negative propaganda made Sun a dangerous proposition. Sun is said to be responsible for skin cancers, wrinkles, and irreparable skin damage. We are encouraged to hide faces behind large rim hats, protect arms with long sleeves and cover the body with high potency SPFs. Now we are so obsessed by sun avoidance that alabaster sun-virgin skin and ghostly white creatures became the health norm.

That's too bad, because without sunlight we cannot thrive. If you don't believe me lock yourself in a cell without windows for a month. You should feel the difference in a day or two and after a week or so you should feel a new wisdom entering your body: sun gives and maintains life. Without it we perish. That's because every cell in the body has sun sensitive photoreceptors, which activate cellular repair, guard blood flow, mitigate digestion, direct energy production and even decide on the mood. That's right. Sun make us energetic, healthy, and beautiful.

Now you have it. Sunlight is just as important as water and air. Every body part responds to sunlight and science verified that numerous conditions can be helped by it. Insomnia, ADHD, SAD, vitiligo, acne, psoriasis, osteoporosis, hypertension, Parkinson's and even dementia respond well to sun therapy. Sunlight kills germs and boosts the immune system.

You may be scratching your head. If sunlight is so good why do doctors and media try to keep us in the dark? Because "they say" it causes melanoma, a deadly skin cancer. Before you rush to double-layer yourself with the highest SPF you find in panic, let's sift through the info jungle and straighten the facts.

There are three main type of skin cancer: basal carcinoma, squamous cell carcinoma, and melanoma. Only the first two can be blamed on the sun. Basal and squamous cell carcinoma are low grade and grow slowly. Their 5-year survival is 100%.[12] Both carcinomas produce local skin crusting and bleeding, but the resulting ugly patch can be removed by a dermatologist in just one session. Squamous cell carcinoma can spread to other tissues. However, it is so slow growing that it takes years of neglect before metastasis occurs. Interestingly both carcinomas can be cured by a photodynamic therapy. If you think that's weird that's likely because mix up healthy exposure with zero exposure. Sunlight can cause harm only if in excess. In moderate quantities it is a great healer. Sun *exposure* is not the same as sun *over*exposure. While sun exposure is good, sun *over*exposure is not. Walking in a tree lined alley is great, frying on a beach isn't.

But what about melanoma? Isn`t melanoma caused by exposure to sunlight? Melanoma is a deadly word. It is the third most common skin cancer leaves clinicians with little treatment success. If it spreads to vital organs the 5-year survival rate gets below 20%.[13] Due to low treatment success, doctors insist on prevention, which is sun avoidance. That's baffling, because melanoma has never been proven to be sun-related. To the contrary, quite a few studies suggest that a moderate sun exposure is highly preventative. Did you know that outdoor workers have the lowest rates? Maybe sunshine is not as scary as it is made to be. Be wiser. Aim for regular healthy exposure. Your body will love it.

There is even a bigger reason to ditch sun-blocking SPFs. SPFs end up in the environment killing our ecosystem. Sunscreens that wash away from the skin, break down to ingredients that are highly toxic to water creatures. SPF by-products kill plankton and coral reefs. As fish food supply and its habitat disappear so is the fish. Birds, and mammals follow. The only way to stop the eco-disaster is to care about the planet and do something about it. If you think that sun rays can burn your skin away, choose shade, not SPFs. Save a few lives. It feels good.

For the ghostly sun virgins I have one more surprise. Did you know that too much sun is *better* than not enough? Studies show that sun *over*exposure has fewer side effects than *under*exposure. Lack of sunlight has been implicated in a whole host of diseases that cost the world 3.3 billion annually. Insufficient sunlight perpetuates depression, insomnia, rheumatic disorders, gout, chronic ulcers, breast, ovarian, colon, and other cancers, multiple sclerosis, osteoporosis, hypertension, asthma, IBD, SLE, thyroiditis, and various infections. Lack of sunlight worsens diabetes, deepens obesity, and increases the risk for melanoma.[14] Do you think that wide-rimed hats, long sleeves, and ocean-killing sunscreens should be part of anyone's health routine?

Infrareds and dance clubs

It is nice to live in a sunny place, but what do you do if you are locked in winter stricken world zone? What if your skies are dark, and snow banks don't melt for three quarters of a year? What if sunny days are scarce and you don't get six month vacation so you can go South? What if your body is chilled to the bone and cold-loving viruses have a blast in your nose?

There may be a solution for that. It is called infrared heat. Although not the same as sunshine, infrared heat is very penetrating and can warm up the body in no time. Infrared heat comes in various sizes, infrared cabins, small heaters, and flat mats. These can fit any space and any budget.

I know that lying on a cozy infrared mat may be more attractive than intense exercise, but I have to mention it here. Exercise is so beneficial to health I cannot leave it out. It not only boosts the BBT, but also nicely reshapes the waist. However you look at it, exercise makes bodies hotter.

Not all types of exercise will do. For thermogenic effect, you need to choose moderate or high intensity activities. Intensity generates heat, watching TV not so much. If you are not up to chasing a soccer ball or madly punching a boxing bag, get creative. Body warming activities are endless. Sign up for a dance class, challenge your friend to a badminton game, or just power walk with your dog. Have lots of fun and get your body fire going!

Chapter summary:

Lifestyle upgrades	Action	Did that!
Cold foods	Memorize & avoid	
Warm foods	Memorize & include	
Sunlight	Schedule moderate exposure	
Infrared sauna or mat	Consider	
Exercise	Make a schedule and follow it	

Chapter 5

Get an exercise boost

Western societies aren't keen on exercising. We know that physical exertion is healthy, but we somehow can't get around doing it. Healthy hearts and strong bones can't persuade us to get up from sofas and chairs, because we have two issues with exercise. It is physically exhausting and does not work as quickly as we want it to. Why bother with months of squats and push-ups when Norvasc can fix blood pressure and Fosamax can mend brittle bones? Why bother with a gym membership if losing weight is as easy as a liposuction.

When I came to North America few decades ago I discovered fitness magazines. Although I never subscribed to them, I picked up a copy or two from a local grocery store. I couldn't help it. My eyes got stuck on alluringly vivid and exceptionally captivating cover photos. I have never seen more sexy bodies than those on the covers.

I peeped through the glossy pages. They were full of great looking athletic physiques advertising exercise routines for specific body parts. Bar bell lifts for a flat belly and squats for strong-looking legs. I got the message. Exercise equals sexy. I joined the gym only to give up a few months later due to lack of results.

The next few years were free of exercise. I did not see any point in it. I wanted a sexy body and I expected exercise to do that. But two months of gym attendance wasn't hassle free. It was time consuming, exertive, and highly upsetting my normal routine. Besides, the payoff in the sexy department was dreadfully delayed.

I never considered exercising for health. In my mind health and exercise had nothing to do with each other. For all health matters I had my doctor. He was the one in charge of dispensing magic pills. I thought health was easy. If broken, all I needed to do is to get my doctor scribble a few words on a prescription pad. A few days of swallowing the miracle tablets and my health would return to normal, at least I thought.

Two decades later I know better. One cannot build health with pills. Funny, but I actually try to master that domain by becoming a physician myself. I was a willing participant of the pill-for-health scheme for over two decades just to realize with horror that it does not work. After my own health started to fail miserably on many fronts I was forced to look at things differently.

Today I know that health and exercise go together like bread and butter. They are inseparable. Strong immune system and sedentary lifestyle don`t mingle together and it does not look like Mother Nature is about to make any changes to her health policy any time soon. You may as well embrace it: exercise is the backbone of the immune system.

I wasn't taught any of this in a medical school. Exercise for strengthening the immune system was a strange concept to me. Doctors don't prescribe Zumba classes. Dance moves and medical curricula somehow don`t go together. Doctors prescribe lab-tested, white-coat approved medication, not some frivolous boogie wiggles. Picture your doctor teaching you that!

Today I exercise, not because I dream of a sexy body (too late for that), but because I know that regular physical exertion can do more for me than a team of medical specialists with a pile of pills. Why bother with anti-inflammatories and anti-pyretics, when a little bit of wild conga can burn the bugs out to begin with. Why bother with sniffles, when a few knee bends and hip wiggles can build the strongest immune system one can dream of. Etch this in your mind: when it comes to health, exercise is not an option. It is a necessity. If you find time to breathe, poop, or brush your teeth, then you for sure can schedule some sweat time.

Exercise has many immune benefits. Here are just eight of them to wet your appetite.

1. It boosts BBT

It is a no brainer. Physical exertion cranks up the body's internal heat. That's why no one turns on the stove before aerobics or wears a fur coat to the gym. Exercise is so thermogenically potent that it can simulate mini-fever. When muscles are at rest they reflect normal resting metabolic rate. However, when they start contracting they may even go into the fever range. Intramuscular probes showed that active muscles increase their core temperature by as much as 1°C (1.8°F). That's a huge metabolic jump for the body. Just imagine how many microbes pack up and go feeling ousted by your thermo-hostile moves.

A sedentary body produces about 70 watts of energy. That's equivalent to a medium power light bulb. A trained athlete can produce 1,400 watts while exercising.[15] That's kind of like a portable heater. No heat-sensitive microbe would put up with such living arrangement.

2. It stops germ germination

Can exercise actually stop the germs in their tracks? Apparently it can! Moderate exercise boasts measurable results. Moderate exertion is highly effective for prevention of common cold. It shortens duration of the illness and in many cases prevents it entirely.[16]

Exercise offers a great protection not only against common cold, but also against many other sniffle- or sneeze-producing viruses. Apparently, exercise effect is so powerful that it can germ-proof the entire respiratory system. Studies confirmed that moderate exercise significantly reduces the incidence of any viral infection of upper respiratory tract.[17] One of the studies tracked two postmenopausal groups of 50 women over a period of two months. The results were compelling. While non-exercisers missed 67 days, women who exercised regularly missed only 32 days from work.[18] Nature is uncompromising. If you won't find time for exercise, you'd better find time for gluey nose, foggy brain, and infectious sneezes.

3. It increases brown fat

Have you ever wondered why body shivers? When the core temperature dips, the body needs to find a way to raise it. Since contracting muscles generate heat, shivering is the fastest way to do so. Thus in case of a chill you can either warm up by doing jumping jacks or wait till the body does it for you. Shivering is kind of an involuntary form of exercise the body is forced into during thermal emergency. Rest assured, when the body warms up, shivering stops.

The role of shivering is not limited to its immediate temperature-lifting effect. Shivering also prepares the body to better deal with cold in the future. Shivering muscles release irisin, a hormone that changes composition of body fat. Irisin initiates fat browning, or in other words converts white fat to brown fat, a process that has long-term thermogenic effect.

Body fat browning has nothing to do with culinary skills. It has nothing to do with burning butter on a frying pan, either. Fat browning is an important biochemical transformation that improves handling winters. Brown fat is heat-producing. Its job is to protect the body from becoming cold. Brown fat is abundant in babies and that's why children don't mind playing in snow for hours. People who lack brown fat are more sensitive to cold. There is a very good chance that your brown fat supply is exhausted if you frequently shiver.[19]

To increase brown fat storage you must boost irisin. To increase irisin you either have to eat more fat, exercise with intensity, or keep on shivering. Either one works, but I'd suggest butter-rich meals intercepted by short sprints here and there. It is highly effective and totally fun.

4. It moderates myokines

Muscles are not just simply a part of a locomotor system. They are also endocrine organs that regulate the immune system. Muscles produce myokines, molecules that tell other systems how to behave. Myokine production varies with exercise intensity thus different type of exercise can evoke a different immune response. In other words, by changing the exercise intensity a person can boost or calm down his immune response. Studies show that while moderate exercise is immune-boosting, prolonged intense exercise is immune-suppressive.[20]

Lack of exercise is yet another story. Sedentary lifestyle and lack of muscular contracture has been strongly correlated with persistent, sterile chronic inflammatory state of the body which in turn causes pain, fatigue, insulin resistance, and cardiovascular diseases.[21] Generally speaking, if you want to live in misery of chronic inflammation, don`t exercise. If you want to be able to fight infections and inflammations you can't stick to excuses. There is no way to weasel yourself out of regular exercise and hope to stay healthy.

5. It increases oxygenation

Did you know that if not the muscles you won't be able to breathe? Although we have many muscles that assist with breathing, there is one king among them: the diaphragm. Not a single muscle can do what the diaphragm does. The diaphragm, a large muscle that spans the thorax between the lungs and the abdomen is the main muscle assisting with respiration. Diaphragmatic movement changes the size of the thorax and by doing so, increases and decreases the lung volume, known to us as breathing. And although everybody thinks it is the lungs that do the breathing, the lungs only diffuse the oxygen. They don't move themselves and need muscles for that. If the thorax is stripped of the muscles, lungs won't work. There will be no inhalation or exhalation.

We breathe oxygen in not only to live, but also to fight infections. Body-made oxygen bombs are highly lethal. They are the number one weapon used against pathogens. Oxygen bombs called reactive oxygen species or ROS are the first line of defense against microbial intruders[22]. They are highly effective and capable of decimating invading microbial colonies in mere seconds.

One of the more powerful ROS is hydrogen peroxide. Hydrogen peroxide is known to consumers as a man-made antiseptic. Few know that it is also the body's own antimicrobial solution. Hydrogen peroxide is spat out by white blood cells when they encounter a pathogen. It stands to reason that a highly effective immune system must have a good supply of oxygen. Low oxygen weakens response to an infection.[23]

Now you have one more reason to ventilate the lungs on the regular basis. Exercise vigorously to turbo-charge the diaphragm and flood the body with oxygen. If you are ill-stricken, can`t exercise and need to stay in bed, at least take a few deep breaths here and there. Even this will make a difference.

6. It propels lymphatics

The role of the diaphragm does not end with the lungs. Besides providing a steady supply of oxygen for the body, it also assists in lymphatic drainage.

Lymphatic system is a network of highways through which the immune cells move about. Under normal circumstances their flow is slow but continuous. The cells travel along the numerous lymphatic paths while scanning for tissues in trouble. Once they find a party of interest, they exit the highway, put up a fight, die, and their remnants get cleared from the circulation. All seem to work fine as long as there isn't an active chronic focus like a rotten tooth or suppurating tonsils. Perpetual battlefields can turn slow flow into congestion.

When the lymphatic system gets gridlocked and the flow is brought to a stop, it resembles traffic jam on LA highways during peak hours. Nothing moves and everything piles up. But unlike LA highways, lymphatic system won't respond to a police crew redirecting the traffic. Instead it will look for some bicep or leg action.

In contrast to blood lymph is not propelled by the heart. Instead, it is propelled by muscles and to keep going, it needs muscular action. It needs calf moves and torso twists to forward smoothly. It is muscular contraction, not some magic push-button that makes the lymph swish around. Have you seen swollen ankles? This beauty attribute can be frequently witnessed on sedentary obstinates. Yes, those who don't move risk sluggish lymph and lymphatic gridlock.

Now is the perfect time to mention the diaphragm. It is an absolute savior for the lymphatic system. Not only it moves all the time (breathing), but its special location makes it extra valuable for the lymphatic circulation. The large muscle is trapped between the lungs and the liver. Exactly this location makes the diaphragm a perpetual lymphatic energizer. With every inhalation the diaphragm moves down and with every exhalation it moves up. The downward movement of the diaphragm pushes the liver and squeezes its juices out and into the lymphatic ducts. This is how the diaphragm moves your lymph and the immune cells that are stuffed in it.

But the diaphragmatic effect varies. It depends on the force and depth of breathing. Gentle and shallow breathing can't squeeze much juice out of the liver therefore, don`t expect leisure walking to whirlwind your fluids. On the other hand, heavy breathing, an effect of heavy exercise can hustle the immune cells around. Studies done on dogs showed that speed of lymphatic fluid parallels exercise intensity. Here are the results: walking increases lymphatic flow by 121%, running increases the flow by 419%.[24]

Now you should have an AHA! moment. Can a chronically mucus-stuffed nose be nothing else, but a sign of a chronically congested lymphatics? Give your nose a break. Move those stagnant muscles! Exercise is a serious natural nose decongestant.

7. It makes sweat

Did you know that sweat cleanses the body? When the body sweats it carries out toxic substances. Sweat detoxifies many harmful substances including heavy metals. Three of them are: arsenic, mercury, lead can either stall or shut down the immune system. Sweat also removes BPA, plastic known for its immune-suppressive properties.

Despite the stigma of wet underarms, disregard laser treatments that destroy the sweat glands. Sweating does your body good. Maybe an anti-perspirant keeps you socially-acceptable, but it also put your immune system at a disadvantage. Be wiser. Hit the gym, and detoxify!

Did you know that pores are not only cooling and detoxifying engines? They also actively carry out battles with germs. Sweat has a full arsenal of anti-microbial tricks.[25] These can fight a whole range of microbes including: *Escherichia coli*, *Enterococcus faecalis* , *Staphylococcus aureus* , and *Candida albicans*.[26] For this reason you shouldn`t be so turned off by clammy hands. After all, they are less microbe-loaded and less infectious than their dry equivalents. Maybe that's why we sweat profusely during fevers. The sweat not only cools, but also has a germicidal effect.

Once you realize the antimicrobial power of sweat, you may be less likely to suppress body secretions and avoid a popular frenzy of self-disinfection. Hygiene is good, but germo-phobia isn't. Over-washing does not make you cleaner. It only scrubs off natural antibiotics and weakens skin resistance against pathogens.

8. It changes genes

Can exercise change who you are? Believe it or not, it can. We have been made to believe that our genes are unchangeable, that once our parents give us a certain set it stays with us for life. Our eye color does not change, so why should anything else that is determined by the DNA? Well, that's an outdated view. Now we know that genes change constantly and respond to the environment as well as the lifestyle. Genes adapt. Whether you are into prolonged sitting or competitive swimming your DNA will reflect that. Over time you will be good at one task, not necessarily the other (wink, wink).

Did you know that even a single session can alter hundreds or even thousands of genes governing the immune system? Research revealed that a four hour yoga class can change 111 genes related to the immune system, while physical conditioning can make changes to more than three thousands of those.[27] Walking or listening to music does not seem to do much. These non-demanding activities change only 38 immune-related genes.[28] As you can see, it is the intense physical exertion not just a leg shuffle that has a deep immune system effect.

What if you don't like exercise

I don't like exercise either. I always thought it should be discretionary and given options I would gladly check off the "sedentary" box. Many people have done that, so why not me. There are only 24 hours in a day. My time is better spent on reading research than on jumping around.

That mindset followed me until I developed major health problems. Only when my health luck ran out I realized that just as I cannot opt out of pooping or breathing, I cannot opt out of being active. Inactivity leads to misery and there is no way to change it. Unfortunately today`s technological advances make everyone a victim of the circumstances. Now even walking is discretionary.

It took me some time to get convinced that despite an apparent option to move, inactivity is detrimental to my health. After much deliberation on how to incorporate exercise in my life I bought a gym membership. But the change wasn't easy. On Monday I would go to the gym, only to revert to my sedentary mode by Wednesday. Apparently I was not meant to be a fitness fanatic.

Rescuing sanity

After multiple failures it finally dawned at me that I suck at structured exercise. It was too repetitive and too monotonous. I could not digest it, but I did not see how I could change it to my liking. One day I made a breakthrough discovery. I like nature, music, and conversations. If I could only turn them into exercise I could have it both ways. So it happened. Conversations turned into chat-walks, music turned to booty-shaping wiggles, and nature watching turned into trail exploring. The results? I got a burden of structured exercise off my shoulders and a few pounds off my hips.

You don`t have to chain yourself to the gym to have a healthy immune system, but you can`t weasel yourself out of physical exertion and expect to fight infections like a pro. If gym turns you off, make a few modifications to your otherwise passive pass-time that you carry on regularly. To get you started I have a few suggestions:

Suggested modifications

To consider	Turn off passive mode	Turn on active mode
Music enjoyment	Listening	Dancing, wiggling, stomping
Biking	Electrical mode	Pedaling mode
Yoga	Meditation mode	Power mode
Gardening	Sniffing flowers	Rearranging soil
Exploring nature	Driving through	Hiking, backpacking, trekking
Dog walking	Stopping for sniffs and pees	Power walking with limited stops
Kinek or VR games	Using console	Using body
Wearable gadgets	Wearing and monitoring	Programming activities and participating in challenges
Swimming pool trips	Wadding, splashing	Swimming, playing

If none of that works, you can always go back to the gym.

Chapter 6

Harness the elements

If you haven't' heard of hydrotherapy, now is a good time to introduce it. Water has been long used as one of the most versatile modality and its powerful effect has been well-known to traditional healers. Today modern clinicians embrace it as well. From studying vaginal douches, sitz baths, and steam saunas, we determined that water can help shrink hemorrhoids, relieve constipation, ease an itch, relax the muscles, lower blood pressure, and even rejuvenate the skin.

Ancient cultures weren't devoid of that knowledge, either. Benefits of hydrotherapy were recorded by ancient Egyptians, Romans, Persian, and Greek civilizations. Water healing properties were enjoyed by both royalties and general public alike. Today hydrotherapy has evolved into a sophisticated medical treatment and continues being used by traditional naturopaths as well as modern occupational therapists, physiotherapists, and sports doctors.

There is a good chance that you have harnessed hydrotherapy already. Many people have, even though they are not aware of it. Icing sore muscles after a sprain or inhaling steam for congested nose is nothing else but a home version of the famous water cure.

Against infections

Hydrotherapy can truly work wonders for the immune system. It is the least expensive, the least time consuming, and the most widely available therapy for the weakened bodies. Very few therapies can do what water can: significantly cut down on frequency of infections. One study done on four thousand participants reported that 30-day cold shower hydrotherapy challenge was able to cut sick days by as much as one third. This is an exceptional outcome and few other therapies come close. So, don't dismiss the power of your shower and let water be your doctor if your goal is to increase productivity, because a simple hot-to-cold switch for one month can reduce work absenteeism by an incredible 29%.[29]

> *Hot to cold hydrotherapy challenge:*
>
> - Commit to minimum 30 consecutive days.
> - Start and continue the shower as warm
> - End the shower with cold water for at least 30 seconds.
> - Keep cold water temperature between 10-12°C.

The 29% is impressive by itself, but when you realize that the above study was not done at any random time, but during the 2014/2015 influenza epidemic, you cannot but marvel at the results. Achieving a statistically significant outcome during such challenging time should make the study the proverbial pot of gold for the immune-compromised.

If cold showers can help with flu, can it help with a cold as well? Spraying yourself with cold water for prevention of a cold may sound illogical, but apparently it works. Although you may not want to face the penetrating chill, a cold shower may not be an unreasonable proposition. Why do I think so? Because a whooping 91% of chronic snifflers have said so. Nine out of ten study participants decided to continue the "painful" practice. They were of the opinion that the health benefits they enjoyed greatly outweigh the discomfort associated with short-lived chill.

One would think that spraying self with frigid droplets would be less popular than moving about among sickly population, but that's not the case. The hydrotherapy experiment had a higher participation rate than the physical exertion study, even though regular exercise was shown to be superior to hydrotherapy in a sniffle curbing battle. Apparently, more people prefer to stick to cold showers than bar bells despite greater benefits of the latter. The exercise study had 35% sick day reduction, while hydrotherapy only 29%.

The reasons for giving preference to water treatment may be twofold. Some people may see exercise as too physically demanding, other individuals may choose hydrotherapy, because it is less time consuming. Figure out which one fits your lifestyle better. There is nothing wrong with considering both. Imagine where your immune system could end up if you do!

How exactly does water boost the immune system?

Researchers have been long interested in this subject. The answers started to emerge in the last twenty years when hydrotherapy experienced a resurgence of scientific interest. The findings are interesting.

Did you know that cold water does not just make you more cold-resistant? It actually increases production of different types of cells involved in the immune response. These include a number of virus-, bacteria- and cancer-fighting weapons such as leukocytes, granulocytes, IL-6, and natural killer cells. These belong to a powerful arsenal that protects the body not only against germs, but also against cancer. That`s right, against cancer as well.

I hope that you've read enough keywords to persuade you to soak your body in a chilling shower and stop cringing your face while imaging a thick frost buildup on your bathroom walls. Fortunately, you don`t have to freeze your butt in a bucket of icy water to boost your fighting armory. The immuno-stimulating effect can be achieved even in temperature of 18°C.[30]

Hydrotherapy has strict rules. Don`t try to fool nature by soaking in a tepid bath in hope for sniffles to go away. When it comes to the immune system only chill-inducing applications work. Too bad that beach vacation never ends up on a doctor's prescription pad. It should, because dipping self in a cooler ocean, or wadding in a cold stream can help the immune system more than a lazy week in bed.

I say warm water should be banned from the sickly! It is true. Warm water is actually immune-suppressive. Studies found out that warm bathing contributes to the reduction of body's fighting power. Warmth reduces the number of antibody-producing cells, as well as the cells that fight cancers.[31] Warm shower may feel good, but in no way should be used as an immune-stimulant. Wait! Don't throw away your water heater as yet. Warm hydrotherapy, although not useful for sniffles, is a great stress reliever. Use it before a job interview. I hope you won`t have sniffles that day.

Can cold shower kill cold germs? No, it cannot. Cold hydrotherapy is not a germicidal. It is a preventative. Preventative means, it needs to be used before, not during an infection. You shouldn't start cold showers when sneezing and dripping mucus from the whiffer, but when you are well. Planning is a great skill. You don't start saving money for retirement at 75 years of age. That's foolish. The same thing applies to cold showers and sniffles. There is a right time for everything, so don't wait till the bugs make a sludge party in your nose. That would be too late for immune-boosting hydrotherapy.

But what if you are in a middle of a head cold right now? Can hydrotherapy be of any use? Yes, it can. Steam inhalation would work great. It can unblock stuffed noses and decongest rattling chests while significantly reducing symptoms of a common cold. But, besides symptomatic reduction don't expect much of other benefits. Steam inhalation won't kill the virus.[32] For that you need to drop a few drops of essential oils in the bowl of hot water. Eucalyptus, thyme, peppermint, rosemary, oregano, and pine have anti-viral properties and are well suited for congested noses and infectious coughs. Keep them handy on your kitchen shelf. You never know when you'd have an urge to save your head from exploding.

Wet socks

Although cold hydrotherapy should not be used during a cold, there is one exception. It is called wet sock therapy. Surprisingly, cold-wetted socks can be used effectively to bring fire back into the body. I am not joking.

Wet sock therapy is an old folk remedy for reviving frozen feet. It is said to stimulate the immune system, reduce aches, eradicate chills, and improve sleep in sick individuals. You may try it for nasal congestion. Apparently it works well for that as well. This is how you do it:

Wet sock instructions:

1. Get a pair of cotton socks and a pair of wool socks. They must be at least 90% cotton and 90% wool, respectively.
2. Soak the foot part of the cotton socks in cold tap water and wring them out thoroughly.
3. Put your feet in hot water. Soak them for a few minutes until they are hot and pink.
4. Dry your feet off and immediately put the socks soaked in cold water. Put on the dry wool socks on top of the wet socks.
5. Go to bed and keep the feet covered through the night. This is a must. The therapy does not work otherwise.

Earthing

Hydrotherapy has been studied extensively for its immune benefits. Now Earth seems to be experiencing a renewed period of interest as initial research suggests huge health-supporting benefits.

Few people have heard of earthing. Earthing, is literally a ground-breaking discovery. An interest in earthing or using Earth for health purposes has soared since first scientific papers on the topic have been published. Earthing is also known under the name "grounding", because in order to receive the benefits one has to be in contact with the ground.

The concept of grounding is not new. Grounding protects our houses from being struck by lightning. This is accomplished by connecting the house electrical network to a metal rod stuck in the ground. Such simple anti-surge insurance works, because both the metal rod and moist earth are good conductors. They are capable of redirecting the lightning charge towards Mother Earth, which has a limitless capacity for absorbing those mean gushes or electrons.

Grounding does not just benefit man-made structures. Humans and any living organisms benefit as well by discharging their unpaired electrons to the ground. I hope you are not confused by that statement. All living organisms use energy and energy requires electrons, but not every one of them ends up being good. Some turn to become free radicals, a nasty kind of electrons known for their violent behaviour.

One cannot escape free radicals. They are everywhere. While a healthy body produces free radicals in smaller amount, an injury, illness, inflammation or infection seriously increases their load. Free radicals are responsible for DNA damage, chronic degeneration, and accelerated aging. Guess what! Grounding neutralizes free radicals. Great! But what does it have to do with the boosting the immune system?

The immune system and body electrical potential are tightly connected. White blood cells maturation and their behaviour is highly dependent on body's voltage and electrical currents in the body.[33] One can say that it is electrical impulses that regulate the immune system.[34] In fact, healthy and unhealthy tissue can be distinguished by its different electrical potential. An injured site carries a positive charge, while a healthy tissue carries a negative one.[35] Once the tissue heals, it returns to its healthy-state negative potential. But add wrong electrical impulse and you can nullify the efforts of the immune system. Grounding prevents misfires by discharging unpaired electrons into the ground.

Grounding, which has an unlimited ability to neutralize bad electrons and supply the good ones, not only can prevent free radical damage, but also help the immune system function better. Grounding improves the odds for a winning the battle with the pathogens. Studies show that it produces measurable differences in the concentrations of white blood cells, cytokines, and other particles involved in the inflammatory response.[36] That's not all. Grounding can make you feel good. It improves sleep, reduces pain and stress, as well as speeds up wound healing.

Are you grounding?

Have you heard a saying "it heals like on a dog", meaning ultra-rapid? The discovery of grounding got me thinking. Maybe it is not the dog, but the shoeless dog's paws that makes all the difference. Maybe it is not about whether a beast or human, but about whether one touches the ground. Maybe we got it all wrong. Could it be that it is our bare feet and not a pile of drugs that should heal us?

If you are not well, ask yourself a question: are you grounding? Are your feet regularly touching grass, sand, or dirt or you neatly pack them up in stylish shoes so that they never mucky themselves or see the daylight? Are you bearfooting from a beach to a backyard or concrete-, stone-, or rubber- yourself away from the Mother Earth?

Going from an apartment to the car, to the office, to the gym, we seem not to have any opportunity to make any contact with the healer beneath us. Shoes, cars, floors, and pavements all cut us off from the ground. Ironically with all the modern improvements, conveniences, and inventions instead of getting healthier we keep on getting sicker. Maybe it is our disconnection from nature that is making us frail. Maybe it is just that simple. Did you know that all the chronic disease we are plagued by nowadays, from heart to cancer to Alzheimer's, are linked to free radical damage and lack of sufficient body counter-protection?

Here is a thought. If you would like your cuts and bruises, inflammations, and infection heal in a hurry or simply "like on a dog" maybe you should have your feet mucked and soiled before you rely on your bed, pillow, and a litany of drugs. The earlier is definitely more fun.

Ok, feet on the ground is great in summer, but what if it is winter, you live in the city or travel for living? Would you choose to stick your hoofs into a snow bank, dangle them out of an office window or drag them behind a scooter? I don't think so. That's painful and not civilized. Here is a different solution: for that you need find an electrical outlet.

If you know that electrons pass freely between conductors, elements that allow current to flow, you won't have to plant your feet in mud any more. To be grounded on the 28th floor all you need to do is to make use of an electrical outlet, which most likely is conveniently located behind your desk. A three-hole electrical outlet is a modern conductor that connects the outdoor ground to your indoor whereabouts via a metal wire. All you need to do is to plug "yourself" into the grounded outlet and your body won't know the difference. You'd be grounded the same way as if you stand directly in the mud. But don't try to poke the outlet holes with a fork or a knife. You will get electrocuted. Only the grounded hole can be used. If you are not sure which one it is, get yourself a grounding kit. It will make your life easier.

Be patient. Grounding does not work like brushing teeth. You just cannot plug yourself for one minute and be good for the rest of the day. Grounding works only while you are connected to the ground. Not before, not after, so to reap the most benefit, ground yourself all the time. Give yourself at least two weeks of non-stop ground action to see tangible benefits. Plug yourself while sleeping, while working on a computer, or watching TV. If weather permits aim to spend maximum time outdoors and walk barefoot wherever possible. In fact, I am writing this paragraph under a tree with my bare feet stuffed in grass patches.

We live in a modern world and for many of us using water and earth for health improvement may sound like an ancient concept. We have high tech medical equipment, potent drugs, and a highly trained team of doctors to do that for us. Why should we use water and earth when no reputable doctor would ever mention it?

There is a good reason to go back to the basics. Water and earth support health, is available to anyone regardless of their financial status, remains free of side effects and is kind to the planet. None of that can be said about modern medical interventions. They may be convenient, but far from good. They manage disease, their access is limited, they are full of side effect, and leave a large footprint behind by polluting waters and damaging the ecosystem. You've heard that your salmon filet is now served with drug residue in it? It is not a joke. We are running out of clean food sources. The reason why our medical system promotes man-made inventions instead of natural solutions is simple: drugs are big bucks.

To do list:

Do what?	Did that!
Daily cold showers	
Wet socks therapy	
Feet on the ground	
Indoor grounding	

Chapter 7

Mind the nutrients

Just like a car mileage depends on the fuel level in its tank, a person's well-being depends on the amount nutrients available to his body. Our bodies must have vitamin and minerals to function. Bones need calcium, the heart needs potassium, and the immune system cannot run without vitamin D.

Luckily you have many options. A billion dollar health food industry offers myriad of choices and plenty of helpful hints. You can't pass a grocery shelf without spotting a nutritional claim and may end up cross-eyed in a million-bottle supplement department. It is not overkill. It is a good business sense. Products boasting "good source of calcium", "good for the heart", "boosts brain power" disappear from the store shelves faster than their plain label counterparts. Food companies know we are nutritionally obsessed and they use our keyword fixation to their profitable advantage.

With all the abundance of nutritional claims and food trucks zooming through highways one would think that malnutrition is not something we should worry about. Malnutrition may exist somewhere else, but not here in North America. Malnutrition is reserved for marasmus-stricken children in Africa or homeless elderly in India, not North American specimen.

North Americans are well off. We are affluent and we are choosey. We eat exactly what we want, when we want, and in any imaginable quantities. There is no way we could be nutrient deficient. We have so much food that we throw it away without a second thought. We are basking in abundance and it shows. We are so well-fed that we tip the scale to the right. Three quarter of us are overweight and many grossly obese. When even an average Joe lugs around leftover calories around his waist it is hard to fathom he could be malnourished.

But looks can be deceiving. That average Joe may have hidden nutrient deficiencies despite visible proof of excess calories. It's because calorie-rich foods are not the same as nutrient-rich foods. One can be thin and well-nourished or fat, but yet short of nutrients. It has been estimated that 95% of Americans do not consume the recommended daily intake of the most important vitamins and minerals.[37] In other words, most of us are nutrient-deficient, and that means we are malnourished.

I bet you don't consider yourself malnourished. You eat well. You take pills. You listen to your doctor. Ok, let's see. Can you tell me what your selenium or zinc levels are? Can you tell me when was the last time your doctor tested you for CoQ10? Can you tell me if your last meal was nutrient-dense or calorie-dense? I can sense a blank stare on your face. I bet you don't know. If you don't know, how can you be sure whether your body has what it needs? You can`t!

Patients seldom ask. Doctors seldom test. The sad truth is that clinicians don't give a much thought about nutrient deficiencies when dealing with symptoms. Few consider join pain, fungus on toes, or recurring infections a nutritional problem. But they all are, without exception. A robust, well-fed body can defy inflammation, guard against infections, and avoid chronic diseases with ease. Unfortunately, instead of boosting the nutritional reserves clinicians prescribe anti-inflammatories, antifungals, or antibiotics. The vicious "get sick, take a pill, get sick again" cycle continues while patients stay poorly fed.

We live in truly backward times. We keep on chasing nutritional claims, but we excuse doctor's nutritional incompetence. We know how important vitamins and minerals are, but we think it is perfectly fine when a doctor makes a diagnosis and recommend a treatment without testing for nutrients first. We will spend all sorts of money on health-promoting supplements, but we are somehow totally convinced that our weak immune system or an autoimmune disease is due to an unfortunate genetic misalignment. Blind leading the blind may be a good description of our health care today.

But being proactive is not an easy task. Try to ask your doctor for a full nutritional panel and he is going to look for the panic button. There is not a single nutritional test that can cover all the nutrients. Moreover, many of these tests are completely foreign to an average doc. Luckily, not every test has to see a doctor's signature. Many tests are accessible to consumers via internet. Online sales make things much easier although not always free from hurdles. Regulations vary from a country to a country, from a state to a state, and from a lab to a lab, restricting what test one can access.

Testing nutritional status

You probably want to know how you score in the nutrient department. That's great. Have a few tests done but don't sweat if you can't find a screen for rubidium or vitamin F. You don't have to chase every vitamin and mineral to get your immune system going. Your immune system can do just fine when it has ample amount of a few key nutrients. Here they are:

Nutrient	Test type	Doctor tested?	On-line kit?
Vitamin D	Blood	Yes	Yes
Vitamin A	Blood	Yes, but unlikely	No
Vitamin C	Urine	No	Yes
Selenium	Hair sample	No	Yes
Zinc	Hair sample	No	Yes
Copper	Hair sample	No	Yes
Iron	Blood	Yes	Yes

Getting the most out of the diet

If you find yourself on a low side of nutrients, look for good quality supplements first. It can quickly boost your body reserves. However, don't attempt to supplement yourself forever. Remember, the reason for malnutrition is not lack of pills but poor diet. Make better choices and you will see the immune system flourish. Start by picking from the list of foods that are rich in immune-specific nutrients. You will find those below.

Vitamin D: Butter, egg yolks, cod liver oil, liver, milk, oatmeal, salmon, sardines, sweet potatoes, cheese.

Vitamin A: Liver, fish liver oil, apricots, asparagus, beet greens, broccoli, cantaloupe, carrots, collards, kale, papaya, peach, pumpkin, red peppers, spinach sweet potato, yellow squash.

Vitamin C: Berries, citrus, asparagus, avocados, beet greens, black currants, grapefruit, lemons, onions, oranges, papaya, green peas, sweet peppers, pineapple, radishes, rose hips, strawberries, tomatoes, watercress.

Selenium: Brazil nuts, brewer`s yeast, broccoli, brown rice, chicken, dairy, garlic, kelp, liver, molasses, onion, salmon, seafood, wheat germ; Be aware that selenium content in food is highly dependent on soil quality.

Zinc: Brewer`s yeast, egg yolks, kelp, lamb, legumes, lima beans, fish, meat, mushroom, pecans, oysters, poultry, pumpkin seeds, sardines, seafood, sunflower seeds.

Copper: Almonds, avocados, barley, beans, beets, blackstrap molasses, broccoli, garlic lentils, liver, mushrooms, nuts, oats, oranges, pecans, radishes, raisins, salmon, seafood, green leafy vegetables.

Iron: Eggs, fish, liver, meat, poultry, green leafy vegetables, almonds, avocados, beets, blackstrap molasses, dates, lima beans, kidney beans, lentils, millet, peaches, pears, prunes, pumpkin, raisins, sesame seeds, watercress.

Fantastic! Now you know what to eat. But before rushing to get any leaf or seed at a random grocery store, consider that nutrient density is not the same across the market. A firm celery stalk bought from a sustainable farm is denser in nutrients than a whittled celery stalk bought on sale at your cheap grocer. Unprocessed oat flakes bought at an organic aisle is more immuno-promoting than a boxed conventional oat cereal. Chicken is not the same as chicken nuggets, blueberries have not much in common with blueberry muffins, and almonds don`t squirt milk. Choose wisely and eat fresh. Leave Franken-foods, food imitations, and processed foods on the shelves.

De- sugar your life

Sugar suppresses the immune system. Lab tests show that that sugar increases inflammatory markers right after it is ingested. Blood glucose spikes are a major contributor to oxidative stress, which over time can ruin the immune system.

Sugar comes in two sources: simple sugars and carbohydrates. The latter are highly deceiving. While sweet things like fruits or candies obviously contain sugar, carbohydrates such as bread and pizza, do not look like sugar and don't taste sweet. But don't get fooled! Every bit of a carb from the innocently looking slice will be broken down into simple sugar once it gets to the stomach. When you sink the teeth into a bun or a muffin, you don't eat a wholesome meal. You eat sugar. From biochemical perspective it makes no difference to the body whether you eat a candy, rice, potatoes, or pears. The digestive system will extract piles of sugar from any of them.

How would you know if you are a sugar junkie? There is a simple test. Look at your naked profile in a mirror. If your stomach sticks out, chances are carbs rule your menu. Truncal obesity is a characteristic sign of carb and sugar overindulgence. Large waist is a hallmark for degenerative physiology and that's not good. Big gut leads to cardiovascular pathology and a weak immune system.

You want to be healthy? Deflate your stomach! Drop your fruit juice and smoothie habit; stay away from pastry shops and refuse junk even if wrapped enticingly. Reduce eat-outs and say no nutrient-questionable foods. Learn how to cook and always choose nutrient-dense ingredients. Factor in organic meats, fatty dairy, organic fruits, nuts and vegetables into your diet. Be picky and choosey. Your immune system will know whether you eat top quality food, or cheap slaps on the go.

Summary:

Do what?	Did that!
Check for nutrient deficiencies	
Plan for sugar and carb reduction	
Set weight loss goal and plan	
Make room for cooking at home	

Chapter 8

Build a sick box

Once you have dealt with nutrient deficiencies expect your body to make a strong turn-around and head towards better health. Removing deficiencies is the key to boosting body vigor. However, in case you fall ill and need an extra boost you can resort to supplement tricks. The ones mentioned below I found to be the most effective.

Supplements can be divided into two categories: one for acute and one for chronic ailments. They are not to be mixed up or substituted, because of the different effect they have on the body. The first category should be used sort of as an emergency kit, when you get sick, not in between. It is meant to rev up the immune system for a short time. The second category contains slow-acting immune-regulators. These are less helpful in an acute contagion, but they are unsurpassed when it comes to regulating and improving the function of the immune system.

To organize yourself properly, have your immune-pills divided into two boxes. One box with pills for sick days (category one) and one for when you are your normal self (category two). Ideally, you alternate between them depending on how you feel. However before you self-medicate, ask your doctor if he sees any contraindications. This may be especially important if you are on prescription medications. Drugs can alter body metabolism and that change can make even the safest supplements highly dangerous. If your doctor says "no" don't just walk away. Always ask "why". It is not uncommon that medical practitioners try to stop patients from using supplements, not because these pills could pose a danger, but because they are either biased against natural medicine or simply lack the knowledge about natural products. A simple "why not?" can clarify things.

Here are my favorite candidates for the "sick box".

Echinacea

Echinacea is number one on the list. It is great for common colds, flus, and sinusitis. Besides helping with upper respiratory troubles Echinacea can also be helpful for herpes, tonsillitis, bladder, and ear infections.

Studies on efficacy of Echinacea for infections vary. A review published in Lancet found that it can prevent common cold in 58% cases and shorten the duration of symptoms by 1 to 4 days.[38] That`s quite impressive. However other studies say it does not work as well.

My clinical experience with Echinacea is positive, although a few factors can make a huge difference as to its effectiveness. Cheap and highly diluted products work poorly, so don't waste your money on dollar store versions. Liquids work better than pills. Tinctures and extracts work faster and are more potent due to their superior absorption rate. Timing also makes a big difference. Echinacea works best at the *onset* of the symptoms, not at the peak or the end of the sniffle journey. Once "ripe" you'd be better off with an antimicrobial, not an immune-stimulant. When your nose runs wild and brain is stuck in a fuzzy land Echinacea may not be sufficient.

Remember to use Echinacea only when sick and only for a short period of time. Echinacea is a potent immune-stimulant, thus prolonged use of the herb may cause immune system overstimulation. Be extra cautious with an autoimmune disease. Echinacea may exacerbate it.

Goldenseal

Hydrastus canadensis, popularly called goldenseal, is a valuable backup herb in case of a more serious microbial invasion. *Hydrastus canadensis* has impressive properties. It was even suggested as an effective treatment in H1N1 flu pandemic. A study from 2011 revealed that the herb strongly inhibits flu viruses as well as activates body`s multiple anti-viral defenses.[39] But *Hydrastus* is not a one trick pony. Besides flu bugs it is also highly effective against several other nasty pathogens including *Staphylococcus aureus*, a bacterium responsible for boils and toxic shock syndrome.[40]

There are a few issues with Goldenseal. It may not be widely available and it may be expensive. The reason behind it is worth noted. Goldenseal has been on an endangered list since 1991. It disappeared partially because of overharvesting and partially due to destruction of its habitat. Thus, don't grab it from a shelf, due to a plain fancy. Consider its endangered status before using it for any infection. If you need to have a similarly potent herbal antimicrobial, give olive leaf a try first.

Olive leaf

Olive leaf is not a new discovery. It has been used for colds and flus for many centuries. The reason why you've never heard of it is because remedying infections with olive is more popular in Mediterranean climate, where the trees grow. Try not to mix up olive leaves with olive oil. Although olive oil has some antimicrobial properties, olive leaf is a completely different animal. While olive oil may be good for warding off bad skin bacteria[41], olive leaf can battle the worst kind of internal havoc.

Olive leaves contain several active constituents capable of killing pathogenic bacteria and blocking viral replication. Because they can eradicate a wide range of microbes, the leaves are excellent for stopping upper respiratory as well gastrointestinal tract infections. Among the bacteria and fungi that bow to the leaves are: *Bacillus cereus, B. subtilis, Staphylococcus aureus, Pseudomonas aeruginosa, Escherichia coli, Klebsiella pneumoniae, Candida albicans*, and *Cryptococcus neoformans*.[42] Olive can also wipe out a litany of hostile viruses including herpes mononucleosis, hepatitis virus, rotavirus, bovine rhinovirus, canine parvovirus, and feline leukemia virus, para-influenza.[43] If you are not sure what bugs you, consider olive leaf. It can fight bacteria, virus, and fungus all at once.

Elderberry

Elderberry, a must for anyone's flu cabinet, also goes also under a more sophisticated name sambucus. Sambucus is an exceptionally potent plant, and can help when other herbs fail. Unlike Echinacea, elderberry is effective at the beginning as well during a well-developed infection, because it has both an immune-stimulatory and direct antimicrobial effects.

Elderberry extract is effective against a wide range of viruses and bacteria. Among the microbes arrested by elderberry are: *Haemophilus influenzae, Staphylococcus aureus, Streptococcus mutans, Haemophilus parainfluenzae, Bacillus cereus, Escherichia coli* and *Pseudomonas aeruginosa.*

Some studies confirmed elderberry's effectiveness, not only as an infection fighter, but also as a convenient preventative. In one study two weeks of prophylactic use of elderberry extract resulted in reduction of the symptoms as well as visible shortening of the cold by 2 days. Elderberry does not have to be taken as a botanical extract. Drinking juice or eating berries is fine too.

No zinc lozenges in the sick box?

Did you notice that your sick box contains only plants? There is a reason for it. Vitamins and minerals are far less effective than herbs for acute sicknesses. Don't get me wrong. They are useful. However, my clinical experience showed that effectiveness of mega-doses of zinc, vitamin A, or vitamin D during an acute illness depended greatly on nutritional reserves of the individual. Those who are helped by zinc lozenges, A or D pills are simply low in those nutrients. Resist TV ads and keep your hands in the pocket when passing pharmacy entrance displays. They are there to bring profits to the seller, far less to you. When your friend swears that zinc lozenges cured his recent cold, chances are that he was simply zinc deficient. Be a good friend. Suggest a more nutritious diet for the poor fellow.

Are you eating out frequently? Are you a vegan? Is your diet limited to a few items? Too bad. After decades of helping patients getting back to health I came to a strong conclusion that restricted diets aren't good for health. People who favor processed foods and restrict quality animal products can't hope for a strong immunity. Poor nutrition isn't compatible with a robust body.

But even when all food groups neatly land on a plate one may end up in a nutritional fiasco. Modern agricultural practices are known to mal-treat plants and animals rendering them a poor source of nutrient and a huge source of toxins. Have you ever wonder why supplement industry is booming? That's why! Everybody eats, 95% are malnourished.

How to evade the fate of everyone? Choose quality foods. Look out for plants that have been grown in nutrient rich soil and animals that have been fed their natural diet. In other words, purchase your food directly from self-sustainable farms or at least pick organic brands in a grocery store. While we are at it, don't forget to load up your cart with quality eggs, dairy and meats. These are great immune builders. Seriously.

Summary of the sick box

Name	Actions, uses
Echinacea	Immuno-stimmulant, use at the beginning of an infection, anti-tumor
Goldenseal	Anti-viral, anti-bacterial actions
Olive leaf	Anti-viral, anti-bacterial, anti-fungal properties
Elderberry	Viral infections

Chapter 9

Jump-start the menu

Now since you have your "sick box" ready you can take a short break. But don't bum around waiting casually for the next flu virus sending you to bed. Instead, stuff your kitchen with antiviral ammunition. Grocery stores abound with immune-protecting bullets. You just need to know what these are. Luckily, the two proven immuno-regulating ingredients are widely accessible and are rather inexpensive. Dairy and oats are the two big guns you may want to keep handy.

Is there something wrong with dairy?

Dairy has received a bad rap in the last few decades. The rumor is that it produces mucus, causes wide-spread lactose intolerance, and its production violates animal welfare. There are many reasons why people choose not to touch dairy. I have formed a strong opinion about dairy during my clinical days and here is my take on it: unless you have been diagnosed with a dairy allergy you should really consider eating the white stuff by the bucket. It is one of the better immune-boosting foods.

Before I go any further, I would like to bring attention to dairy quality. This subject frequently escapes milk debates and causes ongoing confusion among consumers. Yet, things are quite simple: while dairy from healthy cows is healthy for humans, dairy from unhealthy animals does not have such properties. Before including dairy in your daily menu, ensure that butter, yogurt, and kefir you are about to buy, come from grass-fed, humanly treated cows, not from animals standing in their own manure and eating silo by-products. If you buy sick dairy, not only you won't get all the health benefits, but your dollar will continue supporting sick commercial farming. I don't think that's what you have in mind.

Consumers looking for the healthiest dairy versions have one more hurdle to overcome: government bureaucrats. Public servants can spoil even the best intentions of responsible farmers. Some countries and states regulate that all dairy, before it is released to the public, is pasteurized regardless of the source. I understand. Pasteurization makes sense when milk comes from a sick cow and contains pathogens. However, raw milk from a healthy cow should not be treated as a toxin. Unfortunately, bureaucrats don't care. Public protection is big business. Regulations bring lots of money, whether from paperwork, cost of additional procedures, licensing fees, or monopolies that get created as a result.

For the sake of your immune system, avoid pasteurized products like the plague and buy raw whenever possible. Raw milk from a healthy cow has loads of bacteria that support human health. Boiling those away won't make the immune system any stronger. Milk bacteria contribute to increased microbiota in the gut, which directly benefits the immune system. Heat also destroys delicate bonds between proteins, fats, vitamins, and other health-promoting compounds, and by doing so, deactivates them. Moreover, heated milk becomes less digestible and more toxic to the tissues. For example, high heat deactivates enzymes responsible for lactose digestion and leave milk laden with Maillard products. Those can contribute to mineral malabsorption[44], diabetes and kidney disease.[45] Choose your dairy products with care, because your immune system quality parallels the quality of your food choices.

Make whey your friend

Whey comes from milk. Whey is a by-product of milk curdling or a milky substance that gets left behind from cheese production. Whey is a great aid to building a robust body. Studies on whey demonstrate that it is not only good for fending off germs, but is also an effective safeguard against the big "C".

A strong immune system requires strong redox reactions. Redox, the key biochemical process of living organisms, stands for reduction-oxidation. To function well redox require two ingredients: an ample oxygen supply to kill the bugs and good antioxidant supply to prevent oxidative damage to the adjacent cells. Whey provides raw ingredients to facilitate, regulate, and support healthy redox reactions. It does it by supplying proteins that boost glutathione production.[46] Glutathione, a principal antioxidant produced inside the body, deactivates free radicals and maintains healthy levels of vitamin C and E.

Glutathione also plays a role in improving oxygen delivery. It does it by regulating production of nitric oxide, a compound responsible for vasodilation. When capillaries widen they improve tissue oxygenation. Besides facilitating antioxidant production and oxygenation glutathione also participates in DNA repair, protein transport, and enzyme activation. As you can see, not a single body system can function without the presence of glutathione. However, lack of glutathione would be reflected the strongest by poor function of the immune, digestive, and the nervous system.

Whey has a direct ability to boost immunity. One study demonstrated that 600 mg of high quality whey over three months significantly decreased the number of common colds.[47] While only 48 colds were noted in the whey group, the control group suffered 112 colds, which is more than double. Other studies confirmed that whey supplementation can similarly be effective against influenza, because of its antiviral properties.[48] Whey immune-boosting attributes are not limited to infections. Whey has been recently suggested as an effective adjuvant treatment for cancer.[49]

I point to one caution about whey. Raw whey has plenty of lactose. This may pose a problem for some lactose-sensitive people, who may end up with bloated stomachs, gurgling, and diarrhea. The solution is not to avoid whey, but to look for whey isolates. Isolates are completely free of lactose and are safe for lactose intolerant. The only thing you may not be happy about is that isolates are way more expensive. If lactose is your enemy, give isolates a consideration. Maybe keeping your belly calm is worth those few extra isolated bucks.

Where's beta-sitosterol?

Would you believe that breakfast of oats and milk can be better for your immune system than the proverbial apple that keeps a doctor away? Would you fathom that a blob of cottage cheese slapped on organic piece of bread can provide far more immune protection than the store-bought orange juice everyone seems to be hooked on? Myths and habits are hard to break.

Let me introduce beta-sitosterol, a phytochemical that aroused many health maniacs in the recent decade. Beta-sitosterol has many functions. It serves as a precursor to hormones, reduces bad cholesterol, and guards urine flow in men with overgrown prostates. As science discovers its new applications, it is proving that beta-sitosterol and the immune system are inseparable.

Beta-sitosterol exhibits various immune-regulating properties. It normalizes the function of several immunological subgroups as well as their supporting hormones. Studies in pigs showed that beta-sitosterol has anti-inflammatory, anti-neoplasic, anti-pyretic and immune-modulating activity.[50] In plain language it means that it reduces pain, decreases cancer risk, lessens fevers and helps the immune system function optimally. Beta-sitosterol is capable of reversing chronic immune-mediated abnormalities. Two common examples are allergies and rheumatoid arthritis. Beta-sitosterol can also be helpful in serious immune break downs such as in auto-immune diseases, cancers, tuberculosis and chronic viral infections.[51]

Someone has estimated that for a strong immune system we need about two grams of plant sterols a day. Fine, but this is exactly where the problem lies. An average American diet has only 250 milligrams.[52] That's 10% of what's needed to have a robust beta-sitosterol-boosted immune system. Hmm, does your immune system feel like it is also working at 10% capacity?

Beta-sitosterol can be found in edible plants. Among the richest sources are grains, legumes, and nuts. But don't fool yourself. Even vegetarians have a hard time with the goal. They usually reach only 700 mg a day. To give you a perspective you would have to eat 80 apples to get those 2 recommended grams.

Should you then reach for supplements to benefit your health? Should you look out for sitosterol-enriched margarines, yogurts, or cereals to prop up your daily intake? I don't think so. I think that food should be naturally rich in nutrients and those nutrients should be sufficient for boasting good health. If you find food that has been artificially fortified, it is an indication that this particular food does not score well in nutrient density. Fortification is not applied to nutrient-rich, but only to nutrient-poor items. Stay away. Instead, make an effort to find unadulterated variety that is grown in nutrient-rich soil. You will be much better off.

Take all recommendations with a grain of salt. Don't indiscriminately force a nutrient down your throat just because some expert says so. By blindly chasing the 2 gram beta-sitosterol goal you may help your immunity, but at the same time ruin your digestive system. Large quantities of plant sterols can cause indigestion, abdominal discomfort, nausea, and constipation.

Forget the unachievable and potentially gaseously explosive goal. A simple addition of handful of nuts and seeds to your daily menu may do you wonders. Raw peanuts, almonds, walnuts, sunflower or pumpkin seeds are the best immune-supporting choices. If additionally, you can sprout them before eating, the immune system will get a major wave of goose bumps.

Foods rich in whey

- Ricotta cheese
- Goat and cow milk
- Yogurt

Foods rich in beta-sitosterol

- Avocados
- Pistachio nuts
- Almonds
- Macadamia nuts
- Hazelnuts,
- Red lentils
- Pecans
- Walnuts
- Eggs
- Bananas
- Butter
- Pomegranate

Chapter 10

Enhance with adaptogens

Here comes a bummer: being diligent about food choices and having no nutrient deficiencies does not guarantee a perfectly functional immune system. Weakness can happen for other reasons, either due to an ongoing stress, or due to environmental causes. So, if your immune system, despite your best efforts, somehow caves into every cold and flu, it is time to look into adaptogens.

Adaptogens are not fast-acting immune-boosters, like Echinacea. They act slowly, gradually spreading their influence over many related systems. Adaptogens stabilize multiple physiological processes, from sugar metabolism, to blood flow, to responsiveness to stress. They promote whole body homeostasis and should not be confused with immune-stimulants. Adaptogens are not suitable for acute infections. Rather they should be used in-between them. Adaptogens are praised as longevity tonics and are sought after by endurance hunters.

We know several potent adaptogens. Among the most popular are: Asian ginseng (*Panax ginseng*), siberian ginseng (*Eleutherococcus senticosus*), ashwagandha (*Withania somnifera*), licorice (*Glycyrrhiza glabra*), reishi (*Ganoderma ludicum*), rhodiola (*Rhodiola rosea*), schisandra (*Schisandra chinensis*), shiitake (*Lentinula edodes*), and astragalus (*Astragalus membracenus*). They all have body-strengthening effects however, I will focus only on astragalus, schizandra, eleutherococcus, as well as medicinal mushrooms due to their special affinity for the immune system.

Astragalus

Astragalus is an extremely popular herb in Traditional Chinese Medicine. It practically disappears from the shelves during two seasonal changes, when leaves fall and when snow melts, the time when viruses scout for their victims. But don`t confuse it with NyQuil. This small shrub is not for easing the symptoms for the sake of comfort. Its job is to make the body more resilient and unyielding to the elements. Astragalus is prescribed for the weak and sick, especially when there is a need to boost energy, improve circulation and increase resistance to infections.

Western research has praises for astragalus as well. It appears that the herb can significantly help strengthen weak individuals and boost their immune system.[53] It has antiviral properties, which is especially deadly for viruses with upper respiratory tract affinity.[54] [55] Astragalus increases lymphocytes,[56] white blood cells that fight viral infections and cancers. Astragalus seems to be very suitable for people that need enhanced flu, and cold defenses.

Siberian ginseng

Siberian ginseng (*Eleutherococcus senticosus),* another adaptogen native to Asian land is used in Traditional Chinese Medicine to increase the energy of the Spleen, Lungs, and Kidneys. Siberian ginseng tonifies these organs so well, that besides helping the sick, it is frequently sought by high-performance athletes. Eleutherococcus has been proven to boost physical performance as well as to alleviate pain.[57] [58]

Siberian ginseng is also a great general preventive. It has potent immune-modulating properties and offers a solid protection during cold and flu season. One double blind placebo study showed that people who take this herb experienced a drastic increase in the number of immunocompetent cells.[59] Don't think however that the immune-boosting properties of ginseng are limited to flu and cold infections. The herb comes to the rescue even in the most complex cases, where drugs or other herbs perform poorly. These include HIV infection, chronic fatigue syndrome, and autoimmune illnesses such as lupus.[60] With such a wide spectrum of properties ginseng should be considered by people stuck with any type of immune system malfunction.

Schizandra

If you need to astringe the lungs, replenish your Qi or nourish the kidneys you should bring home Schizandra. Schizandra, surprisingly also an Asian herb, excels in treating chronic coughs, spontaneous sweating, and general body weakness. Schizandra, similarly to ginseng, exhibits immune-regulatory properties. It does it by balancing various immune sub-divisions.[61]

Schizandra excels in chronic fatigue. It helps patients overcome post-viral weakness and helps them recover from flu-induced exhaustion. It also reduces prostration due to chronic inflammation. Russian studies found that the herb offers protection from hostile environments and ruthless elements. It makes body resistant against extreme temperatures, the ones that cause heat shock, skin burn, hypothermia, and frostbite. It also protects the body against inflammation, irradiation, and heavy metal intoxication.[62]

Medicinal mushrooms

Medicinal mushrooms are not your white caps or creminis, but exotic varieties capable of potentiating body defences. Medicinal mushrooms are a relatively recent discovery and science is still not able to say with certainty which mushrooms are best for what type of immune problem. Many mushrooms haven't been tested yet, and those who got tested appear to have such incredibly wide range of actions that it is hard to say what they are really good for.

In Traditional Chinese Medicine mushrooms such as reishi, cordyceps, shitake, agaricus, and maitake are considered incredibly precious. They are praised for their tonic properties. In the past they were treasured so deeply that ordinary people were prohibited from using their parts. The mushroom fame spread and in the 20th century western medicine confirmed that ancient Chinese doctors were right. Mushrooms immune-boosting properties have been officially confirmed through recent formal studies.

Now we know that these mushrooms have strong nutritive, anti-inflammatory, and anti-oxidant properties. Their trial applications in inflammatory disorders such as asthma, food allergy, eczema, rheumatoid arthritis, atherosclerosis, diabetes, blood clots, HIV infection, listeriosis, tuberculosis, septic shock, and cancer can be considered a medical success.[63] How do mushrooms do that?

Mushrooms stimulate the immune system by activating robust macrophages and dynamic natural killer cells. These in turn order the release of energetic cytokines, the ones that reduce inflammation. The cytokines visibly downregulate pro-inflammatory markers, the source of stress for doctors and patients alike.

Mushrooms can also enhance battles against infections. Agaricus successfully fights *Streptococcus pneumoniae*[64] and reishi can reduce some resistant bacterial strains known for attacking the skin: *Staphylococcus aureus* - responsible for toxic shock syndrome, *Pityrosporum ovale* - accountable for a disturbing skin discoloration, *Staphylococcus epidermidis* - guilty of forming antiobiotic-resistant biofilm, and *Propionibacterium acnes* - known for aggravating facial pimples. Reishi also has strong antiviral properties. It is effective against HIV, herpes virus, as well as various types of influenza.[65] [66] That's not all. Reishi, together with agaricus and cordiceps, exhibit anti-tumor properties. Some combinations have already been used with success in prophylactics and treatment of various cancers.[67]

Summary of adaptogens

Name	Good for
Astragalus	Frequent infections, chronic cough
Siberian ginseng	Chronic fatigue, chronic viral infections
Schizandra	Chronic fatigue, environmental sensitivity
Reishi	Immune system breakdown

Chapter 11

Invite homeopathy

A huge portion of western clinicians considers homeopathy nothing else but witchcraft. Opponents of homeopathy claim it is useless and believe that whoever uses it must either have something wrong with his head or be a money-greedy charlatan praying on innocent people. In many areas of North America homeopathy is fought with vengeance and even outlawed. Some see it not just a useless fad, but possibly a dangerous practice.

A battle about validity of homeopathy has intensified in the western hemisphere in the last few decades. It looks like homeopathy is losing. Currently no reputable doctor would dare to suggest this unproven sugar pill to a patient. That would constitute a malpractice and may even lead to a license suspension. Peeking outside the regulatory borders just does not pay when a good paycheck is at stake.

Meanwhile in the Eastern hemisphere homeopathy does well and many reputable doctors eagerly prescribe it. Patients love it, because it is cheap, highly effective yet gentle. No one complains about any side effects, except visible improvement in health, surge of energy, and rapid disappearance of annoying symptoms.

Homeopathy flourishes in India and Pakistan. In India alone there are about 200,000 registered homeopathic doctors with 12,000 being added every year.[68] Other countries consider homeopathy a valuable modality as well. Brazil, Chile, Mexico, Switzerland, United Kingdom include homeopathy in their national health systems. Queen Elizabeth has been using it for near a century and she isn't just dabbing in it. She puts full trust in the "witchcraft". She named a homeopathic physician to be her personal doctor. Has she been severely misinformed, confused or her senses got taken over by a Britishly diabolic power? Think for a moment. Something must be working if she hit 91 without clutching a cane.

Homeopathy has been used since 1796. Initially it was tried only by Samuel Hahnemann, a physician that discovered it. But due to its incredible effects, bordering with a miracle, homeopathy spread like a wild fire in a draught stricken countryside. Soon not only Germans were experimenting, but also French and English physicians got fascinated. The fame was difficult to contain as homeopathy seem to excel in curbing plaques and epidemics. It tackled typhus fever in 1813, cholera in 1830s, yellow fever in 1850s, diphtheria in 1860s, influenza pandemic in 1918, and polio in 1950s.

Just to give you a perspective, here is a historical data comparing efficacy of homeopathy with conventional treatment methods.[69]

Epidemics	Mortality with homeopathy	Mortality with conventional tx
Typhus fever	1%	>30%
Cholera	7-10%	40-80%
Yellow fever	6%	50%
Diptheria	16.4%	83.6
Influenza	9%	59%
Polio	No cases of prodromal symptoms developed into polio	None needed to be treated

Today homeopathy is far from the limelight. What happened? The birth of modern pharmacology happened, that's all. 1828 saw a birth of organic chemistry and in 1921 pharmacology was founded. Suddenly there were two competing medical system in place confusing doctors and patients alike. Which one was better, which one was right?

Homeopathy and pharmacology opposed each other, partially due to their focus, partially due to bias of the physicians. Homeopathy and pharmacology stood more contrary than the proverbial cat and dog. They were clashing like political parties before elections. One was based on energetics, the other on chemistry. One aimed to boost the life force, the other focused on suppressing the symptoms. One was widely available and cheap, the other was patentable and thus highly profitable.

Time passed. Profits won. Lobbying money convinced North American governments that homeopathy was quackery and only "science-based" and "evidence-based" medicine was to be used. So it happened. Today few conventionally trained doctors dabble with homeopathy. It is too controversial. It is also difficult for many to imagine that something that does not have a single molecule could have any effect on the body.

I understand. Physicians are trained in chemistry and chemical reactions require molecular interactions. So how can anything work without a single atom? Oh, well, nature could care less about our opinions. It carries on with zero-molecule sunlight visibly browning the skin and changing body's biochemical parameters, zero-molecule thunderstorms turbo-charging rheumatic pains, zero-molecule mistral winds sinking the entire populations into depression, and sub-zero temperatures frostbiting ears and intensifying autoimmune flare-ups. Energetic phenomena surround us, yet somehow lag to be acknowledged by the "educated".

Homeopathy is difficult to grasp even for a willing physician. How do you dose a non-molecular substance? Do you prescribe one unit of energy or send a patient home with a bag of joules? Homeopathy cannot be packed in milligrams. In homeopathy, grams have no meaning. All it matters is how energetic the energy is. What?

Homeopathic remedies are prescribed based on their energetic vitality, or potency. A potency of 6 is small, local, and will act on physical tissue.

A medium potency of 12 works deeper and can regulate biochemical processes. A potency 1,000 acts super- deep and it is capable of smoothing out nervous system kinks.

Homeopathic woes do not end with dosing. There is yet another aspect of homeopathy that confuses the hell out of every clinician. Homeopathy does not need a diagnosis, because it is not prescribed for an ailment. There is no homeopathic remedy for diabetes or sinusitis, yet it is used for those.

Homeopathic prescription is based on symptoms, very detail symptoms. Let me explain. While pharmacies carry just a few painkillers that work for every pain from headache to knee arthritis, a homeopath must have at least thirty remedies just to ease a frontal headache. It is because there is a specific remedy for each specific symptom. There is one remedy for a headache pounding on top of the head, one for a headache showing up before a thunderstorm, one for tightness behind right ear, one for pain from loud noise and one for hammers pounding on the forehead. Mix the symptoms up and you end up with zero results. Crazy, isn't it?

But if you get the symptoms right and get the right remedy you will end up with a miracle. Your headache may disappear in 20 seconds, flu in 20 minutes, and ear infection in one hour. This is insane! But to get such results you need to know homoepathic remedies quite well. With 4,000 remedies stocking shelves it is much easier to prescribe a wrong pill than the right one. It is also much easier to blame homeopathy for its ineffectiveness than a practitioner for his lack of knowledge. Get it?

Homeopathy works, but needs a highly skillful prescriber. When you come across a study claiming its ineffectiveness rest assured that the remedy was prescribed for a medical condition, not for specific symptoms. If we try to assess a new paradigm with old tools, maybe the tools need to be upgraded first before the paradigm is called useless.

Homeopathy works incredibly well for sniffles. A good prescription will work within the proverbial seconds, but for that you need to see an experienced homeopath. Forget about Dr. Google. He does not have enough insight.

Health food stores and pharmacies may offer homeopathic combinations for flu, colds, or sinusitis. These can work in certain situations, but they lack the speed and depth. You can give them a try if you are new to homeopathy, but if you want to venture to single remedies in hope to experience a miracle here is a list of the most common ones with their guiding symptoms. You can give them a try. Use 30CH. This potency is safe for newbies. Don't try to self-prescribe homeopathy for a chronic condition. It won't work. Only a well-seasoned homeopath can tackle the complexity of your body. There is one more thing. Homeopathy works far better if your body is ready for healing. If biochemical and energetic pathways are blocked, don't expect homeopathic miracles. Remember, before homeopathy works, healthy lifestyle is a must.

Homeopathic remedies for sniffles

Aconitum (Acon) – wind shield

When you get that sudden chill from cold Nordic winds in fall or snow blowing on your face during a snowshoeing expedition you would be glad you have Aconitum in your pocket. Aconitum is a wind shield. If you take it right after cold gusts find their way under your jacket, aconitum can stop the chill from turning into nasty sniffles. This is one remedy to always keep at hand, because you never know when Mother Nature decides to have a fit.

Allium cepa (All-c) – onion nose

Allium cepa, a remedy made out of onion, is prescribed for profuse nose drippings of thin watery nature, like those in common colds or allergies. But allium cepa will help only when the mucus coming from the nose is irritating. This remedy won't help bland discharges. An excoriated upper lip can be a good indicator that the drips are sufficiently acrid. Watch for the sniffles stopping outdoors and restarting in a warm room. This would be another good indicator that Allium cepa can work.

Arsenicum (Ars) – cold and fear shivers

Arsenicum helps with weird types of sniffles: when the nose drips water, but feels stuffed. Sneezing that needs Arsenicum, is abundant, but useless in providing any relief. For Arsenicum cold nights feel unbearable. They aggravate all symptoms. In fact, cold is not tolerable in any form. Restlessness and exhaustion is pronounced, so is fear of death. Think of Arsenicum when feeling cold, fidgety, fearful and miserable.

Eupatorium perfoliatum (Eup-perf) – bony breaks

When flu brings severe aches that feel as if bones are breaking Eupatorium perfoliatum may be just the right remedy. Don't discount it for high fevers or freezing chills. It can help with those as well, but to be effective Eupatorium has to have one guiding indicator: symptoms worsen in the morning between 7-9 am. You won't see that phenomenon frequently, because typical flu symptoms get worse in the evening.

Gelsemium (Gels) – dull weakness

Gelsemium is one of the most commonly prescribed flu remedy. It is useful in slow developing symptoms that cause prostration of the body and confusion of the mind. Watch out for progressive heaviness, dullness, and tremulous weakness. Heavy headaches are common, so are droopy eyelids. Gelsemium will work when passing urine eases headaches and resting in warmth improves all the symptoms.

Hepar sulphuris (Hep-sulf) – irritable cheese

When the sickness sensitizes the body to the environment, think of Hepar sulphuris. Hepar sulphuris does not tolerate noises, drafts, smells, and any form of cold. Those make Hepar highly irritable. The remedy works when the sniffles are no longer thin and easy flowing, but turn into thick green mucus smelling like old cheese.

Nux vomica (Nux-v) – bitchy draft

This is another cold-hating remedy that won't tolerate any drafts or breezes. It is highly irritated and snaps at anyone. The foul mood can get triggered by anything, including draft, cold, noise, or bright light. What's specific is that cold dry air will make the nose very stuffy.

Pulsatilla (Puls) – whiny head cold

Pulsatilla works in ripe head colds accompanied by thick, yellow, tenacious discharges from the nose. Pulsatilla may complain of loss of taste and smell, while exhuming offensive breaths without any knowledge. Pulsatilla craves attention and sympathy, sheds tears easily, and desires plenty of hugs due to her insatiable clinginess. In contrast to other remedies, Pulsatila is not opposed to cold drafts. For her cool breezes bring relief and heat makes everything worse.

I hope these few remedies gave you a taste of complexity of homeopathic prescribing. Because every remedy has a different symptom cluster and different personality, homeopathy carries a few hundred of them just to curb the sniffles. If you don't feel confident about self-prescribing, don't force it. The likelihood of failing to prescribe the correct remedy by a beginner is quite high. If you end up with no results, don't shove the remedies out of the window. The remedies work, but not for the symptoms they were given for.

Chapter 12

Work with the gut

When you drool over a cheese-loaded pizza, or you're about to lick a pistachio ice cream the last thing on your mind are your leukocytes and antibodies. The general assumption is that digesting and fighting bugs are two separate things. Not so. Whether you gulp down a steak, potato, or yogurt, your menu choices have a profound impact on how your body handles infections.

You likely heard of gut microflora, a collection of microbes that inhabit the digestive system. That's because the gut is not a sterile strainer separating food from un-digestibles. It is a huge bacterial sack. But that shouldn't make you swallow disinfectant wipes. Gut sterilization won't do anybody any good. Humans need digestive flora for maintaining health.

Gut flora has been a focus of medical research only in the last twenty years, but the idea that the digestive system orchestrates health is not new. The importance of keeping the gut in good working order has been known to natural doctors and body hygienists for a long time. For those practitioners bloating, heartburn, and constipation were obvious hallmarks of ill gut. Not today. Nowadays digestive disorders are so common that they have become normalized. Nobody seems to be perturbed by bloated stomach, irregular bowels, or acid reflux, because flashy TV commercials have convinced us that digestive nuisances can be erased with just one convenient pill. The only problem is that they offer to mask the symptoms while driving the body into a deeper end of ill-health.

Taking care of the gut instead of just the symptoms should be the aim of every health seeker. There is strong indication that gut bacteria influences practically everything in the human body from beauty to mood to smarts. If your skin glows thank the microbes in your gut, if doesn't, think of your digestion before putting any corrective lotion or potion on your anatomy. Bad gut can flare acne blemishes on the face and pop up psoriatic plaque on the elbows. When the worry darkens your life consider that "gut feelings" is not an idle saying. Some gut bacteria have been found responsible for causing anxiety, depression, and mental disorders. Did you know that gut bacteria can influence cognition and memory so strongly that probiotics are now proposed as a treatment for Alzheimer's disease?[70]

Digestive microbiota interacts with both innate and adaptive immunity and its disruption can cause breakdown of defenses leading to immune-compromise and autoimmune diseases.[71] Studies point out that probiotics, can reverse many types of immune-related diseases.[72] Fecal transplants containing colonies of good bacteria are now being suggested as a viable cure for chronic inflammatory diseases existing outside the colon, like MS, insulin resistance, fibromyalgia, chronic fatigue, Parkinson's and autism.[73]

What does gut have to do with the sniffles?

The immune system is intimately tied to gut health, specifically quality of the gut flora. Research suggests that intestinal flora not only protects the gut, but also cross-talks with the immune system. Microbial communities exert a huge effect on the body defenses. For example, inflammatory and autoimmune markers appear in direct proportion to gut flora composition. The gut can even mitigate upper respiratory tract infections. Studies showed that gut flora improvement can lead to decreased incidence and severity of respiratory illnesses.

How do good bugs fight bad bugs? If you imagine good bugs fighting bad bugs with swords and grenades you may be a tad too far in your daydreaming. Good bacteria do not pull out automatic weapons and ultrasonic jets to prove their point, but fight their battles by using four different methods.

1. Competition for nutrients; good guys can "steal" food from bad guys
2. Direct chemical inhibition; good guys "poop out" substances that inhibit or directly kill pathogens

3. Competitive binding; good guys act as bouncers. They prevent the bad guys from getting into a space where they can settle and form a colony

4. Production of cytokines; good guys talk directly to the immune system asking it to produce pro- and anti-inflammatory cytokines, war- or peace- making tools, depending on the need

Anything specific for sniffles?

Detail studies on the role of probiotics in viral diseases are still ongoing. But even with incomplete information the research suggests that gut flora may have several different anti-viral tricks. Their application varies for different viruses. For example, the gut flora uses one of its by-products lactic acid to suppress HIV virus,[74] but flu virus is ousted by activation of viral antibodies and inflammasomes.[75]

Gut flora importance in viral illnesses cannot be overstated. Studies on mice confirmed that microbiota is vital even in case of flu virus. Specifically, the flora prevents flu virus replication.[76] One animal study made an interesting observation. When mice suffering from flu were given an antibiotic they ended up with an *increased* viral load in the lungs. That's because antibiotics killed off good bacteria, which were needed to fight the flu. Basically, you can translate it this way: lack of good bacteria leads to lack of immunity to fight influenza, or the stronger the gut flora the weaker the flu. Whether the bacteria protects humans against flu the same way as it is in the mice we are yet to discover, but we have already confirmed that probiotic supplementation can be an effective for both the treatment, as well as prevention of many types of respiratory tract infections.

Would you stop blaming the flu virus already!

Influenza is said to be one of the deadliest infections, yet in-depth studies showed, that it is not the flu virus that is deadly, but the flu sequela. The worst case scenarios happen to flu-infected individuals that have low immune system. These tend to develop nasty secondary bacterial or fungal infections. If death occurs it is usually from raging inflammation that accompanies the second infection and not from the presence of the flu virus that initiated the sequela. This is where good gut flora comes in. It lowers host damage by buffering inflammation and quickly restoring immune system balance. In other words, gut bacteria can prevent inflammation from becoming lethal and by doing so reduce deaths from influenza infection.[77]

I need to mention that the secondary infection does not require getting infected with a new pathogenic strain. Many pathogenic bacteria and fungi co-exist with a normal microbiota and appear non-threatening if the good-bad microbial balance is maintained. However, the moment good gut bacteria is compromised, opportunistic pathogens proliferate. They will exploit an impaired host immune system when the protective flora is decimated.[78]

Research on human microbiota is complicated. There are about 100 trillion microbes living in and on our bodies. That's about 10 microbes for every human cell! Oops! That means we are more bacteria than ourselves! The gut alone is estimated to host about 1,000 bacterial species, many of which we haven't started studying yet. So far we don't have sufficient data to conclude on the role of probiotics in common colds. However, initial research suggests that probiotics likely have a direct influence over sniffling frequency. One study found that a three month supplementation of probiotics decreased common cold incidence by 18%. Unfortunately the study could not say the same about longer periods. So far, the speculation is that probiotics can help with common colds, but for the answer on which ones we should use we still have to wait.[79]

How to preserve good flora

Your grandma said "eat your vegetables!" and she was right. That's because vegetables are excellent source of fibre, scrumptious food for the good bacteria. Showering the gut daily with heaps of soft fibrous pre-biotics is a sure way to keep the gut flora happy.[80] A grocery cart neatly stacked with onions, leeks, artichokes, dandelion greens, bananas, and garlic is your top immune system allay.

Did you know that vegetables are not the only pre-biotic foods? Grains, such as wheat, are also a good source. However, before you marry Wheaties for breakfast, know that eating wheat can have drawbacks. First, wheat is a carbohydrate and overeating on carbs leads to obesity, Secondly, many people are gluten and gliadin sensitive. Gluten and gliadin are wheat proteins shown to negatively impact gut ecology in many individuals. Thirdly, commercial wheat products are loaded with glyphosate, a herbicide that kills off good gut bacteria.[81] Due to the above wheat and wheat products can actually cancel out their pro-biotic benefits and instead cause immune system demise through contributing to inflammatory obesity, disrupting digestion, and decimating good flora.

Here is a thought: how about you let go off wheat for a while and see what happens? Going wheat-less may grow into a remarkable nutritional discovery for folks who are immunocompromised, stuck with a bloated stomach, and in constant disagreement with a bathroom scale. If you are up for the challenge, mark your calendar for the next three months and give it a try. Be fiercely prepared, because the challenge can be surprisingly difficult. Wheat can be addictive and cause withdrawal symptoms. If you have wheat cravings or feeling unsatisfied without it, persist. Eventually, things will normalize.

When I proposed a wheat-less diet to few patients of mine they looked at me with utmost disbelief. They could not fathom a day without buns, rolls, or pasta. Polish guys could not see past sandwiches, Italian ladies insisted on serving spaghetti, and Caribbean families felt lost without rotis. Regardless where you came from I assure you, you CAN live without wheat. Reorganizing your menu is a matter of your will, not your cultural background. So put your excuses aside and mark three wheat-free months. Only after completing the challenge you can judge whether your effort made any difference to your gut, scale, or nose. You decide what happens next.

While on the challenge don't forget to add probiotics. They will considerably boost the gut microbes. However, I suggest loading up on fermented foods rather than pills. Fermented foods beat many probiotic pills by quality, quantity, availability and cost. Kefir, kimchi, kombucha, kvass, lassi, miso, natto, pickles, sauerkraut, sour cream, soy sauce, tempeh, and yogurt are examples of fermented foods cherished across the globe. Get some of those.

But before picking up random picklies from a store shelf, know that many commercially available products do not provide gut benefits. Read labels. Sneaky manufacturers use vinegar to mimic the fermented food taste without the hassle of fermenting. Natural fermentation takes time and is complicated, not something that contributes to quick profits. When you see "vinegar" on the back label, skip the product altogether.

While reading labels watch out for the word "pasteurized." Pasteurization is designed to kill off pathogens. The problem is however, that heat does not distinguish between good or bad microbes. If your grocery cart is full of pasteurized produce you may as well assume that it is useless for your gut.

If you can't get unpasteurized dairy, see if you can spot something that at least has some value to your immune system. For example, yogurt fermented with *Lactobacillus delbrueckii* has been shown to reduce the risk of catching cold in the healthy elderly.[82] A yogurt made with *Lactobacillus brevis was* proven to lower incidence of flu in school children.[83] Not into yogurt? Then pick up fermented Korean cabbage instead. It has heaps of *Lactobacillus plantarum,* which provided 100% protection against influenza virus in mouse studies.[84]

How not to kill off your immune system

I hope it is clear by now that well-inhabited gut flora preclude iron-strong immunity and that the immune system will fail without gut support. Having said that I also hope that in the very near future every doctor, every internist, and every immune specialist will put a great deal of emphasis on building health-promoting good microbiota, instead of stuffing patients with antibiotics, luring them to gobble up anti-inflammatory pills, and having them extend arms for immune-boosting injections. The reason why so many people suffer from low immune system today is not the lack of health tools, but massive misinformation and deceptive health leadership. Did you know that 75% of Americans say they eat healthy[85], yet their health is systematically declining? It's because many regularly destroy good gut microbiota without being aware of doing so.

Let's take ill-stricken individuals. Many of them faithfully follow advice of the authorities, eat according to the food pyramid, take prescription drugs daily, and adhere to safety standards only to see their health vanish in the air near retirement. Think for a minute. Should they not be super-healthy if they follow what the doctor ordered?

Beware! Not everything that "experts" endorse as safe and health-promoting, is indeed so. Don`t follow trends blindly, because everyone else falls for them. We are not in an era of massive genetic misalignment, DNA mis-coding of some sort, or unfortunate circumstances that render us all ill. We are in the era of massive health mismanagement equally affecting public and health professionals. It is time to look at those "lifesaving" prescriptions, those "beneficial" agri-chemicals, and those salutary public safety practices with a critical eye as they pose a threat not only to the gut microbiota, but also to life in general.

Are you ever wondering why despite billions of dollars pouring into medical research we are fatter, weaker, and sicker? That's because our society is programmed to normalize harmful practices without much criticism. Eating junk, popping pills, staying inactive, and wasting self on entertainment is nothing abnormal in America. It is how millions of people lead their lives. Unless a miracle happens, consumers invest responsibly, corporations value morals before profits, politicians put public interest before counting votes, and journalists exclusively tell the truth, don't expect things to change any time soon. Your journey towards better health will remain futile unless YOU start reading the fine print and expand your knowledge beyond mass media.

The world of deception is vast and convoluted and it has a direct effect on your gut flora and the immune system. Below you will find three out of many common gut insults you may be unknowingly subject to.

1. *Prescription drugs*

   I don't have to look too far. Remember famous drug Vioxx, marketed as a miraculous immune-altering anti-inflammatory drug that "accidentally" killed 60,000 people in less than five years, more or less the number of US soldiers that vanished in the entire 20-year long Vietnam War?

   It is not a secret that America loves meds. Everyone seems to need a pill for something whether heartburn, allergy, joint pains, or sleep. But meds have immune consequences, because gut flora composition changes according to drugs people ingest.[86] Even innocent contraceptive pills have gut-altering effect, so do corticosteroids, as well as anti-inflammatories that we love so much.[87] All drugs have a potential to wreak havoc to the flora however, one type of medication renders the biggest destruction to the good bacteria: antibiotics, which sadly, we pop like candies. In 2014 alone US patients filled out 266.1 million antibiotics courses with at least 30% of them being completely unnecessary.[88]

   What can you do about it? Be mindful. Minimize medication use. Focus on prevention and try to remedy minor issues with home methods first. Only when absolutely necessary resort to prescription drugs and stay on them for the shortest possible time. Find a cooperative doctor that understands cumulative implications of medication, not just signs of common short-term side effects.

2. *Agri-chemicals*

Commercial agriculture destroys life. You won't find a commercial farmer that does not use toxic pesticides, herbicides, fungicides, and nematicides on his crops. Noxious agri-chemicals are an inseparable part of commercial agriculture today, even though they cause an irreparable damage to the neighboring ecosystems. A question may pop in your head: why does the government allow it? It is all about money. The profits are so lucrative to both the farmer and the government that they silence any health concerns.

Glyphosate, a herbicide that you likely consume with every bite is suspected to be a major health hazard to people and the environment. Glyphosate was invented to facilitate mass production of crops and make commercial farmers' lives easier, but independent research indicates that its costs to humans and the planet may by far be outweighing the benefits. While Europe puts forward an effort to completely ban the carcinogenic[89] demon, unaware North Americans happily gobble it up by the bucket.[90]

Glyphosate, the main ingredient in a herbicide popularly known as Roundup, is one of the more toxic and controversial products used today. Glyphosate, which is a mainstay of commercial agriculture, has been implicated in several lethal diseases from kidney failure[91] to Parkinson`s disease[92]. Recently a new concerned emerged over the ability of glyphosate to alter gut microbiota. Glyphosate has been shown to inhibit replication of beneficial flora and increase the ratio of pathogenic to beneficial bacteria in the gut.[93]

Glyphosate is sprayed on corn, cereals such as barley, wheat, and oats, oilseed rape, legumes including lentils, garbanzos, and soybeans, sunflower, and potatoes. That means glyphosate is in your breakfast bowl, take out sandwiches and nachos, pasta dishes, salad dressings, and popular crunchy snacks that you love so much. The estimated contribution of this herbicide to dysfunctional immune system may be extreme due to its widespread use on food crops.

What can you do about it? Be aware. Suspect that any commercially grown crop carries glyphosate residue. Since herbicide information doesn't show up on the label, you can't rely on it to pick your produce. For that reason, I suggest avoiding *all* commercially grown produce and focusing on organically grown food instead. Better yet, do your own research on pesticide residue for specific brands. Some brands have been deceptively marketed as organic (with all the right stickers), even though they contain shockingly high herbicide levels (!). Also avoid all non-organic meats and dairy. Commercially grown animals are fed with cheap grain and legume by-products. Their meat, organs, and bones are known to contain glyphosate. PS. Cooking does not destroy agri-chemicals.

3. *Public safety measures*

Surprise, surprise! Not everything that the authorities stand for is good for the public. Those who follow news may be aware that many guidelines and regulations that were put forward under the guise of public protection turned out to have a different motive and also a different effect than "intended". From heart-destroying fen-phen to mismanagement of Flint water and the current obesity-promoting food pyramid we all have either witnessed or experienced the disasters coming from deviant policies.

Treatment of drinking water with chlorine and fluoride is another example of those initiatives. Both treatments are guaranteed by the government as safe and necessary whether to remove water-born pathogens or to improve dental health. However, in-depth research should make you a tad suspicious.

First of all, both chorine and fluoride have antimicrobial properties and that means they have antibiotic-like action. This is where your immune system should object. Systematic destruction of gut flora is the number one cause behind dysfunctional immune system. Yep. Chlorine is a disinfectant and that thing may float in your tap water. Chlorine is one of the most effective and cheapest bactericidal we know. A popular house-disinfectant Clorox is nothing else but diluted chlorine. Besides reducing gut flora population, chlorine is also blamed for increased free radical load, cardiovascular damage, growth retardation, breast, bladder and rectum cancers.[94] Swimming classes anyone?

The damage caused by fluoride is not all that different from chlorine's. Fluoride has been found to inactivate enzymes, speed up the aging process, increase the incidence of cancer and tumor growth, cause genetic damage, and disrupt the immune system.[95]

Fluoride may be in tap water as well as many dental products promoted by health authorities.

Fluoridation of water, a practice that is pushed onto North Americans for its dental benefits somehow did not gain popularity in other countries. 99% of western continental Europe has rejected, banned, or stopped fluoridation not due to lack of concerns over European teeth, but due to massive environmental, health, legal, or ethical concerns.[96]

What can you do about it? Minimize chlorine and fluoride exposure. Install purification system to eliminate drinking water contamination. Consider installing a shower filter. 66% of chlorine absorption occurs during taking showers through lungs and skin. Avoid chlorinated swimming pools. Ditch fluoridated toothpaste and fluoride-containing mouth cosmetics and switch to non-fluoride tooth cleaning options. And for the future sake of your immune system... do your research before putting blind trust in policies.

Gut flora summary

Do what?	Did that!
Eat two cups of fibrous vegetables daily	
Go wheat free for three months	
Use naturally fermented product every day	
Aim for a medication-free life	
Choose organic produce	
Install shower filter	
Install water purification system	
Use fluoride-free products	

Chapter 13

Test for hidden causes

It is great to have a sense of a direction, but better yet is to confirm that your hunches are right. For that we have tests. Every patient knows that doctors seldom prescribe without writing a lab requisition first. The only trouble is that labs are not used to discover the *causes* behind the patient's problem. They are to confirm the diagnosis and make out a prognosis. To illustrate, doctors test *whether* one has infection or not, but not *why* the immune system isn't spontaneously resolving it. Doctors test *how many* white blood cells are in a sample, but not *why* the immune system isn't producing enough. No one can bring the body to health without first discovering what it needs, and that's why North Americans have a little bit of a dilemma: despite widespread pharmaceutical use, nobody seems to be achieving the pinnacle of health.

Yet, finding why the immune system fails is not difficult. There are many cause-detecting screens on the market. The only problem is to find a clinician that has a clue about those. Conventionally trained practitioners rarely do, because the body milieu, nutritional, and environmental influences on health aren't emphasized in medical textbooks. As a result both your doctor and your pharmacist may try to banish sniffles in a suppressive way, not because it is good for you, but because that's the way they were taught.

Symptoms are not body mistakes and there is a reason why you have them. Try to resist the urge to conceal them with decongestants, fever reducers, and cough suppressants. They may be inconvenient but they have a function. They make body milieu more hostile to germs (fever) and detoxify the tissue from the bugs and their waste (mucus, cough). Unless you are in a life threatening situation suppressive treatment should be your last aim.

There is a better way to strengthen your body than to continue spending your last few dollars on 4-hour relief pharmaceutical goodies forever. It is called "find your body's weak spots." Look for nutrient deficiencies, imbalanced gut flora, chronic inflammation, or insufficient hormones.

Below is a short list of the most useful tests to help you with the above. Don't be surprised if some tests are familiar to your doctor. They may be, but their interpretation as presented in this book likely isn't. That means your doctor can order them for you, but probably won't resort to unconventional analysis. Don't sweat too much if your doctor won't cooperate, because you can get these tests on line without ever requiring his signature.

1. Do you have chronic inflammation?

While everyone is blaming germs for beating down the immune system, few know that their own body can inflict a much bigger damage to it. Chronic inflammation, which is so common in our society, can insidiously wipe off any strength from the defenses while over time leaving an Armageddon of destruction behind. Chronic inflammation uses an incredible amount of nutrients and energetic reserves giving nothing except a mega dose of harmful free radicals in return. Free radicals prolong upper respiratory tract infections and suppress immune response to viruses.[97] Moreover, oxidative damage which comes from free radicals [98] has been implicated in premature aging and development of multiple chronic diseases. The last thing you should aspire to is to walk about with a decade-old inflammation.

Do you have hidden chronic inflammation? Unfortunately, you can't tell by looking in the mirror. For that you need to pull up your latest blood work and look up WBC. WBC stands for white blood cell count and it is one of the most common tests performed by the labs. WBC is used by every single doctor and appears practically on every single lab report. It is used to detect pathology such as infection or cancer.

But your doctor won't use WBC to determine your inflammatory burden or health status. Such thing would be out of his scope. He can only raise his eyebrows when WBC shoots above 11 or darts below 4. Such high or low numbers would warn that some sort of illness is forming, which may include a major infection, autoimmune disease, leukemia or a troubling immunodeficiency. Since there is no immediate danger to the body when WBCs are within the range, any number between 4 and 11 is considered normal and is left alone. Patients with WBC between 4 and 11 are told they are fine and they have no pathology. But "normal" does not mean healthy.

Let me give you an example. Sedentary lifestyle is normal, but it is far from healthy. Watching TV for 2 hours daily is normal, but for sure won't prolong your life. So is the case with lab ranges. You can live for a long time when numbers hide within the ranges, but they don't mean you are well. They only mean your body isn't ripe for a medical intervention, whether drugs, corrective procedure, surgery, or radiation.

Despite the medical consensus you should not leave your numbers as that. After tracking thousands of patients I realized that WBC consistently poking above 6 correlate with persistent hidden inflammation. This is in contrast to conventional doctors that consider those numbers "healthy" and insist that symptoms such as bloated stomach, spiking blood pressure, stiffness, chronic fatigue, and higher cholesterol are either random or hereditary. Just saying: look at WBC number yourself. You may have another "aha" moment.

Better yet, see the copies of your blood work from the last 5 years. When WBC keep on locking above 6 it is time to put down the body's inflammatory flames. That does not mean you have to fill out a prescription for anti-inflammatory pills. Stay away from those. They don't address the causes and won't restore your health. Their only job is to suppress inflammation, which is the body's natural response to an injury. Address the injury and inflammation will go away by itself. The fastest way to do that is to start avoiding all processed foods and restoring the bowel flora. Sometimes it is that mind-bogglingly simple.

WBC is not the only test that can measure inflammation. hsCRP is another inflammatory screen you may want to look into. hsCRP is not a common lab test so don`t expect every clinician to be familiar with it. hsCRP is most frequently ordered by heart specialists to assess cardiac risk for the patient. Chances are that unless you are under a cardiologists care you have never had your hsCRP tested.

hsCRP has a different range than WBC. Unlike WBC, hsCRP graces low numbers. In hsCRP 1 or 1.5 is good. It means low or no inflammation. But let 3 or more show up and it will make any cardiologist worry. It indicates significant inflammation and an increased risk for heart disease.

When interpreting hsCRP you have to be very cautious. The parameter is highly temperamental and it registers a spike even from a slight infection. Don`t panic if you see 7 or 9. The spike may be due to a minor nuisance. While an odd high hsCRP number may pop up from a tooth or bladder infection, don`t ignore when it is constantly up. Keep your hsCRP un-inflamed: below 3, and ideally below 2.

2. Does stress drag you down?

The immune system does not work in isolation. It constantly responds to signals coming from different parts of the body. Stress and stressors are a big part of the feedback loop. Stress can activate segments of the immune system modifying its short and long-term functions. For example, a short-lived stress, such as a seasonal flu typically boosts the defenses, while chronic stress, such as habitual overworking, drags the immune system down. Chronic stress not only contributes to more frequent infections, but can also lead to development of autoimmune disorders and malignancies.

Stressful lifestyle is a normal part of the North American culture. Everyone feels some sort of stress on a daily basis, whether at home, work or in a relationship. And it is not a matter whether you do or not, but whether the amount of stress you encounter negatively impacts your physiology.

Wet hands, dry mouth, buzzing in head are familiar symptoms of feeling under pressure. While acute stress is easy to spot, chronic stress is elusive. When the body keeps on being traumatized it eventually gives up. It stops fighting. Racing heart, sweating of palms, and drying throat disappear and the body resorts to a new solution. It calls cortisol for help.

Cortisol, the main stress hormone normally fluctuates according to its circadian schedule. Its usual small quantities do the body a whole lot of good. But when cortisol gets overproduced the immune system suffers. This is what happens when the body is under chronic stress.

It is hard to tell whether the body has too much of cortisol merely by looking at a face. However, there are other signs that can provide valuable clues. Frequent infections, easy irritability, a stomach bulge, low sex drive, chipping teeth, or high blood pressure may all be due to cortisol excess. In such cases you want to refer to your cortisol numbers.

The most accurate test for cortisol is four-point saliva test, which measures the hormone at four different times of the day: one upon waking, one at noon, one in the late afternoon and finally one the evening. These points after being connected yield a curve that demonstrates cortisol behavior. When the cortisol curve runs high it is a sure sign that the body is caving under the burden of chronic stress. If this is the case, you need to reduce stress before attempting to repair the immune system. Without that first step, boosting the immune system can prove to be futile.

While ordering the saliva cortisol test you may also want to add another test: DHEA. It will give you additional information about the severity of the situation and the necessity of hormonal supplementation. DHEA is a hormone and also responds to chronic stress, but not in the same way cortisol does. When your results come back and you see that both DHEA and cortisol are high, it means that the body still copes with chronic stress, but at a high cost to the immune system. However, when both hormones are down, it is a signal that the body lost its fighting powers. Low cortisol and low DHEA go with chronic fatigue and severely compromised immune system. In such a case a temporary supplementation of DHEA may be necessary. Since DHEA is a steroid you will need to contact your health care provider for guidance on use and dosage. Don`t take any hormones without the consent of a knowledgeable health care practitioner.

3. How robustly cholesterol-ed are you?

Cholesterol has been given a bad reputation due to its implication in heart disease. But correlation does not mean causation. If you bought into this confusion, you are not alone. The entire medical community did. Medical professionals keep on blaming cholesterol, even though there has never any definite proof that high cholesterol is to blame. In fact, it looks like the opposite may be true. New studies suggest that the practice of lowering cholesterol not only does not help the heart, but inadvertently hurts the rest of the body. Low cholesterol is linked to depression, antisocial behaviour, hemorrhaging stroke, adrenal fatigue, poor digestion, and low immune system among other effects.

Did you know that biochemical cholesterol is the backbone of the immune system and that individuals with the low numbers have a hard time fighting germs? Statistics show that the lower total cholesterol the higher mortality from infections and parasites. For example, total cholesterol below 150 mg/dL (4 mmol/L) correlates with more than 1% of deaths from infections. This is a huge number. Meanwhile total cholesterol above 220 mg/dL (5.7 mmol/L) has close to zero casualties.[99] That's not all. Low cholesterol is so detrimental to the immune system that it makes cancers deadlier.[100]

My clinical experience confirmed the above. Patients with cholesterol below 150 mg/dL (4 mmol/L) kept on making appointments for runny noses, head colds, and sinus troubles. They were cursed by frequent infections, recurring colds, never-ending flus, and had overall lack of body defenses. Exactly those patients made their cardiologists, who commented on their "perfect cholesterol numbers," happy. Unfortunately, outside of the cardiac department the "perfect numbers" were not turning into perfect health, but into low-grade fever, malaise, and body aches. Sometimes life throws you a tough choice between "perfect numbers" and perfect health. Make good judgments.

Total cholesterol is important, but good cholesterol is even more vital. Good cholesterol, known also as HDL is another number you should be ogling on the lab reports. Is your HDL below 40 mg/dL (1.0 mmol/L)? That's not good. Super-low HDL number is bad news, because it diminishes body's robustness. When HDL is up your body is "unbreakable", but when it goes down so does the body verve. Low HDL shows up in chronic inflammation[101] and in the unfortunates with compromised immune system. Where should your HDL be? Somewhere above 70 mg/dL (1.8 mmol/L). How can you perk it up? Through magic of exercise!

4. Are you short of nutrients?

No one can thrive without adequate nutrient reserves, because just like a car needs fuel for driving, one needs nutrients to live. Poor nutrition means poor health. And that's why it is not surprising that in today's era of junk food, aka foods low in nutrients, everyone seems to have at least one chronic ailment. If most chronic symptoms are due to low nutrients, wouldn't it make sense to start from boosting nutrition instead of prescribing symptomatic treatments? It does not make sense to send a car that only ran out of gas to a mechanic. Neither does it make sense to prescribe drugs without checking nutrients first. Sadly, current medical system firmly turns a blind eye on patients' menus while eagerly drugging them according to the established protocols. It is not uncommon that a doctor would write a prescription for a high blood pressure pill while patient's hypertension originated from lack of magnesium, or he would give a drug that lowers cholesterol, which shot up due to low antioxidants.

The immune system is not any different than the cardiovascular system. It also relies on vitamins and minerals. Does your immune system have what it takes? If you don't know, you should check your nutrient levels. Unfortunately, there isn't just one test that covers all the nutrients. Vitamins are best tested from blood. Minerals need a hair sample.

Although the body relies on thousands of different nutrient types, you don't have to test them all to be in good health. The immune system will be happy with ample reserves of just six of them.

The most crucial nutrient for the immune system is vitamin D. Low levels correlate with poor defenses. Inadequate vitamin D is found in people, who are prone to flu, viral upper respiratory tract infections,[102] autoimmune diseases[103], and cancers.[104] Don't be surprised to find out that even though few organs and systems can function without it you may have never been tested for it. Vitamin D test is not a part of regular physical. If you can't find vitamin D screen on your latest blood work, ensure it gets added during your next clinic appointment. Otherwise you can get a test kit on line.

Low levels can be remedied by supplementation, but before you reach for a pill, ask yourself a question: *why* did you end up with a deficiency in the first place. Are you eating a low fat diet, avoiding outdoors, or overusing sunscreens? Correct the causes before treating the end effect. Pills are convenient, but they are never a good permanent solution. Besides, chances are that vitamin D deficiency is accompanied by deficits of other fat-soluble vitamins: A, E, and K. Only by improving the diet you can address them all.

There are five minerals that the immune system thrives on: selenium, sulfur, iron, zinc and copper. Although iron can be measured in blood, other minerals cannot be tested that way. For accuracy they require hair analysis.

Hair mineral levels correlate quite well with body reserves. That's why thick lush hair is a natural attribute of a robust body. Elderly and malnourished don't swish their thick locks around. Instead, they present limp and thinning coiffures. Treat poor hair as a nutritional warning. Did you know that thinning hair is a well-known symptom of iron-deficiency anemia?

Where can you get hair analysis done? Don't count on your conventionally trained physician. He likely never heard of it. Instead, look for a licensed health care provider focusing in nutrition. He may be able to help. If you don't know any, there is always an on-line order. You will find a link to an accredited medical laboratory specializing in hair analysis on our website.

5. Are you laden with toxins?

Unless you have eaten salmonella-laden eggs, chewed on poison ivy leaves, or drank some laundry detergent, your doctor may not consider testing you for toxicity. For a doctor to suspect toxicity he has to see obvious symptoms and get a lab confirmation. That's great, but what do you do when none of that is possible? What do you do when symptoms creep up so slowly that you can barely notice it? What if the symptoms are so vague that they are mistaken for a different problem? What if the substance in question is not very well known? What if...

I once had a case of a patient with vague symptoms: fatigue, achiness, spiking blood pressure, headaches, and constipation. The family doctor resorted to giving him a mild blood pressure pill and suggesting drinking more water, none of which helped. The patient ended up in my clinic and we screened for heavy metal toxicity. Lo and behold the results were shocking. The patient had a major long-standing lead poisoning from small but consistent exposure at work.

We are surrounded by substances that we don't suspect to cause health issues. We inhale them, eat them, and use them on a daily basis. And it is true that they don't pose a threat to us when sporadically bumped into, however daily exposure over time may unexpectedly lead to a serious health breakdown.

You may think that toxicity does not apply to you, because you live carefully, but think again. Do you use aluminum foil for cooking or eat out frequently? Do you eat grains sprayed with glyphosate? Do you charcoal your meats? Do you eat large fish or bottom feeders? Do you live in a basement? Do you live in a city? Do you use air fresheners? Do you take long steamy showers? Do you use dry cleaners? Do you use cosmetics? Do you take recreational drugs or prescription drugs? The list can go on.

Modern world exposes us to a myriad of chemicals. It is impossible not to run into them. You use them when you shampoo your hair or clean your shoes. You eat them when you order a burger or brush your teeth. You inhale them when you smoke or splash yourself with perfume. Over time they can have dire consequences on health. The problem is that there aren`t many tests to screen for *cumulative* toxicity of commonly occurring chemicals.

This is where hair analysis comes in handy again. Hair analysis won't show pesticide or plastic accumulation in your body, but at least it can detect heavy metal buildup. Heavy metals, especially arsenic, aluminum, and cadmium can shut down the immune system. These metals are lurking everywhere. They are in cooking foil, batteries, cosmetics, pharmaceuticals, even rice, salt, apple juice, and infant formulas. If your hair results show metal accumulation, you need to deal with it first, before the immune system gets a lift.

Hair analysis is great for detection of heavy metals, but this is where its magic ends. Microbial toxins and environmental toxins cannot be identified from hair. Unfortunately, there aren't many tests for the above. The ones that can be purchased on line are listed on our website.

6. How good is your gut flora?

Testing for gut microbiota is not a routine practice. Standard stool tests are limited to checking for parasites, such as salmonella, tapeworm, or entamoeba. They don't check for opportunistic gut bacteria and yeast that alter microbiota. So, when you ask your doctor for gut microbiota test he may believe you want to check for common parasites. Explain your needs properly otherwise you may end up paying for a useless test.

Several laboratories perform the gut screens. Look around for the best option, because the quality and accessibility of the tests vary by country, state, and the regulatory framework. A comprehensive microbial test should screen for beneficial as well as harmful microorganisms and their balance. It should also give suggestions on how to improve the gut composition.

Summary of tests:

Test what	Name	Sample	Where?
Inflammation	WBC	Blood	Any clinician, on line
Inflammation	hsCRP	Blood	Some MDs, on line
Stress	Cortisol, DHEA	Saliva	On line
Heavy metals	Hair analysis	Hair	On line
Environmental or endogenous toxicity	Changeable	Various	On line, check our web site for updates
Intestinal flora balance	Gut microbiome	Stool	On line

Chapter 14

Try home remedies

According to surveys home remedies are the most preferred way to treat sniffles. From neti-pot to chicken soup, snifflers share their positive experiences on internet. Some swear by vitamin C, some give orange juice a credit. Some praise oregano for miracles, some are cheering vodka with pepper. Out of myriad of possibilities, which one should you choose? Which one could cure your ails?

Don't overthink it. Choosing one remedy over another should be more a matter of your personal preference rather than scientific evidence. Home remedies are not backed up by solid studies, because of their low profitability. Why study something that doesn't benefit the sponsor's pocket? Home remedies are cheap, widely available, and cannot be patented. Exactly for that reason scientists don't swarm around them. There is little profit to be made on salt water gargle.

Don't get confused. Lack of studies does not mean home remedies are ineffective. They are just not studied well. Despite the drawback give some a try. Maybe one or two will become your all-time favorite. Here are 12 most popular remedies for chest and nose indispositions.

- Garlic
- Ginger
- Lemon + honey
- Chicken soup
- Oregano oil
- Baking soda
- Thyme
- Warmed wine with cloves
- Cinnamon
- Apple cider vinegar
- Salt water gargle
- Black pepper

Stick this list on your fridge. When your head gets fuzzy and brain does not work, you will be glad you have this simple checklist in front of you.

Chapter 15

Enjoy iron strong immune system

Garbage in, garbage out. This popular saying isn't just limited to computer databases. It also applies to the immune system. A healthy body does not happen in a vacuum. It is created and maintained by a healthy lifestyle. For most a malfunctioning immune system has nothing to do with genetic misfortune, but a lot to do a faulty self-care.

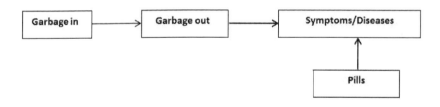

Chronic ailments and pill dependence is an unfortunate effect of our medical system that scores very low on teaching good lifestyle habits and very high on prescribing drugs. Notice that standard prescriptions do not cure the ailments, but treat the dangers and discomforts stemming from existing diseases. Antibiotics don't cure weak immune systems. They only kill the opportunistic bacteria that found a suitable host.

Pills won't make you healthy, strong, symptom and disease free. To be that you need a solid self-care routine that does not require a prescription pad, secret ingredients, vague rituals or membership fees.

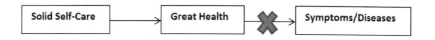

If you want perfectly working antibodies, functional membranes, and wicked white blood cells you need give the body what it needs. It does not need a magic potion in a syringe, sterile environment, or a pile of pills to thrive. It only needs five ingredients. Adopt them and you will greatly increase your chances for staying healthy, sniffle free, and immune-strong for good.

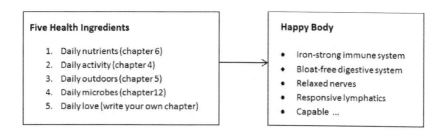

You get the point. Health is a skill, not a pill. DrD.

References

[1] Common cold. Retrieved April 4, 2017 from Wikipedia.com;
https://en.wikipedia.org/wiki/Common_cold

[2] R. Eccles (2002). An Explanation for the Seasonality of Acute Upper Respiratory Tract Viral Infections. *Acta Otolaryngol 2002; 122: 183–191.*
http://www.airguardmedical.com/html/content/Eccles%20R_2002.pdf

[3] Influenza. Retrieved April 4, 2017 from Wikipedia.com;
https://en.wikipedia.org/wiki/Influenza

[4] Leading internal analgesic tablet brands in the United States in 2017, based on sales. Retrieved 10 April 2017 from Statista, The Statistics Portal;
https://www.statista.com/statistics/194510/leading-us-analgesic-tablet-brands-in-2013-based-on-sales/

[5] Plaisance K, Kudaravalli S, Wasserman S, Levine M, Mackowiak P. (2000). Effect of antipyretic therapy on the duration of illness in experimental influenza A, Shigella sonnei, and Rickettsia rickettsii infections. *Pharmacotherapy. 2000 Dec;20(12):1417-22.* PMID: 11130213;
https://www.ncbi.nlm.nih.gov/pubmed/11130213

[6] Laura Hudgings, MD Kelsberg, Gary Sarah Safranek, MLIS (2004). Do antipyretics prolong febrile illness? *J Fam Pract. 2004 January; 53(1):55-71.*
http://www.mdedge.com/jfponline/article/60191/do-antipyretics-prolong-febrile-illness

[7] Ralf Kleef and E. Dieter Hager (2000-2013). Fever, Pyrogens and Cancer. *Madame Curie Bioscience Database* https://www.ncbi.nlm.nih.gov/books/NBK6084/

[8] Hyperthermia in Cancer Treatment. Retrieved 20 April 2017 from National Cancer Institute. https://www.cancer.gov/about-cancer/treatment/types/surgery/hyperthermia-fact-sheet

[9] Ralf Kleef and E. Dieter Hager (2000-2013). Fever, Pyrogens and Cancer. *Madame Curie Bioscience Database* https://www.ncbi.nlm.nih.gov/books/NBK6084/

[10] Dr. Sircus (2013). Hyperthermia with Far-Infrared for Cancer and Pain. Retrieved 5 May 2017 from DrSircus.com; http://drsircus.com/light-heat/hyperthermia-far-infrared-cancer-pain/

[11] Ibid

[12] Survival statistics for non-melanoma skin cancer. Retrieved May 15, 2017 from Canadian Cancer Society. http://www.cancer.ca/en/cancer-information/cancer-type/skin-non-melanoma/prognosis-and-survival/survival-statistics/?region=on

[13] Melanoma: Statistics (2016). Retrieved May 15, 2017 from Cancer.Net.

https://www.cancer.net/cancer-types/melanoma/statistics

[14] M. Nathaniel Mead (2008). Benefits of Sunlight: A Bright Spot for Human. *Environ Health Perspect. 2008 Apr; 116(4): A160–A167.*PMCID: PMC2290997; https://www.ncbi.nlm.nih.gov/pmc/articles/PMC2290997/

[15] C. Bruce Wenger (1999). Exercise and Core Temperature. *US Army Research Institute of Environmental Medicine* http://www.dtic.mil/dtic/tr/fulltext/u2/a377492.pdf

[16] Hyun Kun Lee, In Hong Hwang, Soo Young Kim, corresponding author and Se Young Pyo (2014). The Effect of Exercise on Prevention of the Common Cold: A Meta-Analysis of Randomized Controlled Trial Studies. *Korean J Fam Med. 2014 May; 35(3): 119–126.* doi: 10.4082/kjfm.2014.35.3.119; PMCID: PMC4040429. https://www.ncbi.nlm.nih.gov/pmc/articles/PMC4040429/

[17] Stephen A. Martin, Brandt D. Pence, and Jeffrey A. Woods (2009). Exercise and Respiratory Tract Viral Infections. *Exerc Sport Sci Rev. 2009 Oct; 37(4): 157–164.* doi: 10.1097/JES.0b013e3181b7b57b; PMCID: PMC2803113. https://www.ncbi.nlm.nih.gov/pmc/articles/PMC2803113/

[18] Barrett B, Hayney MS, Muller D, Rakel D, Ward A, Obasi CN, Brown R, Zhang Z, Zgierska A, Gern J, West R, Ewers T, Barlow S, Gassman M, Coe CL. (2012). Meditation or exercise for preventing acute respiratory infection: a randomized controlled trial. *Ann Fam Med. 2012 Jul-Aug;10(4):337-46.* doi: 10.1370/afm.1376; PMID: 22778122. https://www.ncbi.nlm.nih.gov/pubmed/22778122

[19] Svenia Schnyder and Christoph Handschin (2015). Skeletal muscle as an endocrine organ: PGC-1α, myokines and exercise. *Bone. 2015 Nov; 80: 115–125.* doi: 10.1016/j.bone.2015.02.008; PMCID: PMC4657151. https://www.ncbi.nlm.nih.gov/pmc/articles/PMC4657151/

[20]Stephen A. Martin, Brandt D. Pence, and Jeffrey A. Woods (2009). Exercise and Respiratory Tract Viral Infections. *Exerc Sport Sci Rev. 2009 Oct; 37(4): 157–164.* doi: 10.1097/JES.0b013e3181b7b57b; PMCID: PMC2803113. https://www.ncbi.nlm.nih.gov/pmc/articles/PMC2803113/

[21] Svenia Schnyder and Christoph Handschin (2015). Skeletal muscle as an endocrine organ: PGC-1α, myokines and exercise. *Bone. 2015 Nov; 80: 115–125.* doi: 10.1016/j.bone.2015.02.008; PMCID: PMC4657151. https://www.ncbi.nlm.nih.gov/pmc/articles/PMC4657151/

[22] David A. Wink, Harry B. Hines, Robert Y. S. Cheng, Christopher H. Switzer, Wilmarie Flores-Santana, Michael P. Vitek, Lisa A. Ridnour, and Carol A. Colton J Leukoc (2011). Nitric oxide and redox mechanisms in the immune response *Biol. 2011 Jun; 89(6): 873–891.* doi: 10.1189/jlb.1010550; PMCID: PMC3100761. https://www.ncbi.nlm.nih.gov/pmc/articles/PMC3100761/

[23] Fatma Vatansever, Wanessa C.M.A. de Melo, Pinar Avci, Daniela Vecchio, Magesh Sadasivam, Asheesh Gupta, Rakkiyappan Chandran, Mahdi Karimi,

Nivaldo A Parizotto, Rui Yin, George P Tegos, and Michael R Hamblin (2014). Antimicrobial strategies centered around reactive oxygen species - bactericidal antibiotics, photodynamic therapy and beyond. *FEMS Microbiol Rev. 2013 Nov; 37(6): 955–989.* doi: 10.1111/1574-6976.12026; PMCID: PMC3791156. https://www.ncbi.nlm.nih.gov/pmc/articles/PMC3791156/

[24] Desai P1, Williams AG Jr, Prajapati P, Downey HF (2010). Lymph flow in instrumented dogs varies with exercise intensity. *Lymphat Res Biol. 2010 Sep;8(3):143-8.* doi: 10.1089/lrb.2009.0029; PMID: 20863266. https://www.ncbi.nlm.nih.gov/pubmed/20863266

[25] Deborah Josefson (2001). Bacteria killer found in sweat. *BMJ. 2001 Nov 24; 323(7323): 1206.*PMCID: PMC1173041. https://www.ncbi.nlm.nih.gov/pmc/articles/PMC1173041/

[26] ibid

[27] Maléne E Lindholm, et al. (2016). The Impact of Endurance Training on Human Skeletal Muscle Memory, Global Isoform Expression and Novel Transcripts. doi: 10.1371/journal.pgen.1006294. http://thescienceexplorer.com/brain-and-body/endurance-training-changes-gene-activity

[28] Carolyn Gregoire (2013). Yoga Associated With Gene Expression In Immune Cells, Study Finds Retrieved May 10, 2017 from HuffingtonPost http://www.huffingtonpost.com/2013/04/24/yoga-immune-system-genetic-_n_3141008.html

[29] Geert A. Buijze, Inger N. Sierevelt, Bas C. J. M. van der Heijden, Marcel G. Dijkgraaf, and Monique H. W. Frings-Dresen (2016). The Effect of Cold Showering on Health and Work: A Randomized Controlled Trial. *PLoS One. 2016; 11(9): e0161749.* doi: 10.1371/journal.pone.0161749; PMCID: PMC5025014. https://www.ncbi.nlm.nih.gov/pmc/articles/PMC5025014/

[30] A Mooventhan and L Nivethitha (2014). Scientific Evidence-Based Effects of Hydrotherapy on Various Systems of the Body. *N Am J Med Sci. 2014 May; 6(5): 199–209.*doi: 10.4103/1947-2714.132935; PMCID: PMC4049052. https://www.ncbi.nlm.nih.gov/pmc/articles/PMC4049052/

[31] ibid

[32] Ophir D, Elad Y. (1987). Effects of steam inhalation on nasal patency and nasal symptoms in patients with the common cold. *Am J Otolaryngol. 1987 May-Jun;8(3):149-53.* PMID: 3303983. https://www.ncbi.nlm.nih.gov/pubmed/3303983

[33] Biophysics of BCEC. Retrieved May 11, 2017 from http://www.iabc.readywebsites.com/page/page/623959.htm

[34] Eva Sundman and Peder S. Olofsson corresponding author. (2014). Neural control of the immune system. *Adv Physiol Educ. 2014 Jun; 38(2): 135–139.* doi: 10.1152/advan.00094.2013; PMCID: PMC4056170. https://www.ncbi.nlm.nih.gov/pmc/articles/PMC4056170/

[35] Biophysics of BCEC. Retrieved May 11, 2017 from http://www.iabc.readywebsites.com/page/page/623959.htm

[36] James L Oschman, Gaétan Chevalier, and Richard Brown (2015). The effects of grounding (earthing) on inflammation, the immune response, wound healing, and prevention and treatment of chronic inflammatory and autoimmune diseases. *J Inflamm Res. 2015; 8: 83–96.* doi: 10.2147/JIR.S69656; PMCID: PMC4378297. https://www.ncbi.nlm.nih.gov/pmc/articles/PMC4378297/

[37] How much is too much? Appendix B: vitamin and mineral deficiencies in the U.S. (2014). Retrieved May 13, 2017 from http://www.ewg.org/research/how-much-is-too-much/appendix-b-vitamin-and-mineral-deficiencies-us

[38] Steven D. Ehrlich, NMD. Echinacea. Retrieved 14 May 2017 from University of Maryland Medical Centre http://umm.edu/health/medical/altmed/herb/echinacea

[39] Cecil CE, Davis JM, Cech NB, Laster SM (2011). Inhibition of H1N1 influenza A virus growth and induction of inflammatory mediators by the isoquinoline alkaloid berberine and extracts of goldenseal (Hydrastis canadensis). *Int Immunopharmacol. 2011 Nov;11(11):1706-14.* doi: 10.1016/j.intimp.2011.06.002; PMID: 21683808. https://www.ncbi.nlm.nih.gov/pubmed/21683808

[40] Keivan A. Ettefagh, Johnna T. Burns, Hiyas A. Junio, Glenn W. Kaatz, and Nadja B. Cech (2011). Goldenseal (Hydrastis canadensis L.) extracts synergistically enhance the antibacterial activity of berberine via efflux pump inhibition. *Planta Med. 2011 May; 77(8): 835–840.* doi: 10.1055/s-0030-1250606; PMCID: PMC3100400. https://www.ncbi.nlm.nih.gov/pmc/articles/PMC3100400/

[41] Cicerale S, Lucas LJ, Keast RS. (2011). Antimicrobial, antioxidant and anti-inflammatory phenolic activities in extra virgin olive oil. *Curr Opin Biotechnol. 2012 Apr;23(2):129-35.* doi: 10.1016/j.copbio.2011.09.006. PMID: 22000808. https://www.ncbi.nlm.nih.gov/pubmed/22000808

[42] Pereira AP, Ferreira IC, Marcelino F, Valentão P, Andrade PB, Seabra R, Estevinho L, Bento A, Pereira JA (2007). Phenolic compounds and antimicrobial activity of olive (Olea europaea L. Cv. Cobrançosa) leaves. *Molecules. 2007 May 26;12(5):1153-62.* PMID: 17873849. https://www.ncbi.nlm.nih.gov/pubmed/17873849

[43] Syed Haris Omar (2010). Oleuropein in Olive and its Pharmacological Effects. *Sci Pharm. 2010 Apr-Jun; 78(2): 133–154.* doi: 10.3797/scipharm.0912-18; PMCID: PMC3002804. https://www.ncbi.nlm.nih.gov/pmc/articles/PMC3002804/

[44] Nahid Tamanna and Niaz Mahmood (2015). Food Processing and Maillard Reaction Products: Effect on Human Health and Nutrition. *International Journal of Food Science Volume 2015 (2015), Article ID 526762.* doi.org/10.1155/2015/526762. https://www.hindawi.com/journals/ijfs/2015/526762/

45 P. F. FoxT. Uniacke-LoweP. L. H. McSweeneyJ. A. O'Mahony. Heat-Induced Changes in Milk. *Dairy Chemistry and Biochemistry pp 345-375.* doi.org/10.1007/978-3-319-14892-2_9. https://link.springer.com/chapter/10.1007/978-3-319-14892-2_9

46 Lothian JB, Grey V, Lands LC.(2006). Effect of whey protein to modulate immune response in children with atopic asthma *Int J Food Sci Nutr. 2006 May-Jun;57(3-4):204-11.* doi: 10.1080/09637480600738294; PMID: 17127471. https://www.ncbi.nlm.nih.gov/pubmed/17127471

47 Vitetta L, Coulson S, Beck SL, Gramotnev H, Du S, Lewis S (2013). The clinical efficacy of a bovine lactoferrin/whey protein Ig-rich fraction (Lf/IgF) for the common cold: a double blind randomized study. *Complement Ther Med. 2013 Jun;21(3):164-71.* doi: 10.1016/j.ctim.2012.12.006; PMID: 23642947. https://www.ncbi.nlm.nih.gov/pubmed/23642947

48 Soad H Taha,corresponding author Mona A Mehrez, Mahmoud Z Sitohy, Abdel Gawad I Abou Dawood, Mahmoud M Abd-El Hamid, and Walid H Kilany (2010). Effectiveness of esterified whey proteins fractions against Egyptian Lethal Avian Influenza A (H5N1). *Virol J. 2010; 7: 330.* doi: 10.1186/1743-422X-7-330; PMCID: PMC2998487. https://www.ncbi.nlm.nih.gov/pmc/articles/PMC2998487/

49 Bounous G (2000). Whey protein concentrate (WPC) and glutathione modulation in cancer treatment. *Anticancer Res. 2000 Nov-Dec;20(6C):4785-92.* PMID: 11205219. https://www.ncbi.nlm.nih.gov/pubmed/11205219

50 Fraile L, Crisci E, Córdoba L, Navarro MA, Osada J, Montoya M (2012). Immunomodulatory properties of beta-sitosterol in pig immune responses. *Int Immunopharmacol. 2012 Jul;13(3):316-21.* doi: 10.1016/j.intimp.2012.04.017; PMID: 22595193. https://www.ncbi.nlm.nih.gov/pubmed/22595193

51 Bouic PJ, Lamprecht JH (1999). Plant sterols and sterolins: a review of their immune-modulating properties. Altern Med Rev. 1999 Jun;4(3):170-7. PMID: 10383481. https://www.ncbi.nlm.nih.gov/pubmed/10383481

52 Marye Audet. What Foods Are High in Plant Sterols? Retieved 18 May 2017 from LovetoKnow http://herbs.lovetoknow.com/What_Foods_are_High_in_Plant_Sterols

53 Chinese Herb: Huang Qi (Astragalus), Radix Astragali Membranacei. Rerieved 18 May 2017 from SacredLotus https://www.sacredlotus.com/go/chinese-herbs/substance/huang-qi-astragalus

54 Chuan Zou, Guobin Su, Yuchi Wu, Fuhua Lu, Wei Mao, and Xusheng Liu (2013). Astragalus in the Prevention of Upper Respiratory Tract Infection in Children with Nephrotic Syndrome: Evidence-Based Clinical Practice. *Evid Based Complement Alternat Med. 2013; 2013: 352130.* doi: 10.1155/2013/352130; PMCID: PMC3638577. https://www.ncbi.nlm.nih.gov/pmc/articles/PMC3638577/

[55] Auwalu Yusuf Abdullahi, Sanpha Kallon, Xingang Yu, Yongliang Zhang, Guoqing Li (2016). Vaccination with Astragalus and Ginseng Polysaccharides Improves Immune Response of Chickens against H5N1 Avian Influenza Virus. *Biomed Res Int. 2016; 2016: 1510264.* doi: 10.1155/2016/1510264; PMCID: PMC5002477. https://www.ncbi.nlm.nih.gov/pmc/articles/PMC5002477/

[56] James Meschino. Astragalus: and Immune Support. Retrieved May 20, 2017 from MeschinoHealth http://meschinohealth.com/article/astragalus-and-immune-support/

[57] Ci Wu Jia – Eleutherococcus senticosus root – "Siberian Ginseng". Retrieved May 20, 2017 from ChineseHerbalMedicine http://chineseherbinfo.com/815/

[58] Siberian Ginseng Benefits. Retrieved May 21, 2017 from HerbWisdom. http://www.herbwisdom.com/herb-ginseng-russian.html

[59] Bohn B, Nebe CT, Birr C (1987). Flow-cytometric studies with eleutherococcus senticosus extract as an immunomodulatory agent. *Arzneimittelforschung. 1987 Oct;37(10):1193-6.* PMID: 2963645. https://www.ncbi.nlm.nih.gov/pubmed/2963645

[60] Siberian Ginseng Benefits. Retrieved May 21, 2017 from HerbWisdom http://www.herbwisdom.com/herb-ginseng-russian.html

[61] Lin RD, Mao YW, Leu SJ, Huang CY, Lee MH. (2011). The immuno-regulatory effects of Schisandra chinensis and its constituents on human monocytic leukemia cells. *Molecules. 2011 Jun 10;16(6):4836-49.* doi: 10.3390/molecules16064836; PMID: 21666550. https://www.ncbi.nlm.nih.gov/pubmed/21666550

[62] Panossian A, Wikman G. (2008). Pharmacology of Schisandra chinensis Bail.: an overview of Russian research and uses in medicine. *J Ethnopharmacol. 2008 Jul 23;118(2):183-212.* doi: 10.1016/j.jep.2008.04.020; PMID: 18515024. https://www.ncbi.nlm.nih.gov/pubmed/18515024

[63] Cristina Lull, Harry J. Wichers, and Huub F. J. Savelkoul (2005). Antiinflammatory and Immunomodulating Properties of Fungal Metabolites. *Mediators Inflamm. 2005 Jun 9; 2005(2): 63–80.* doi: 10.1155/MI.2005.63; PMCID: PMC1160565. https://www.ncbi.nlm.nih.gov/pmc/articles/PMC1160565/

[64] Bernardshaw S, Johnson E, Hetland G.(2005). An extract of the mushroom Agaricus blazei Murill administered orally protects against systemic Streptococcus pneumoniae infection in mice. *Scand J Immunol. 2005 Oct;62(4):393-8.* doi: 10.1111/j.1365-3083.2005.01667.x; PMID: 16253127. https://www.ncbi.nlm.nih.gov/pubmed/16253127

[65] Ulrike Lindequist, Timo H. J. Niedermeyer, and Wolf-Dieter Jülich (2005). The Pharmacological Potential of Mushrooms. *Evid Based Complement Alternat Med. 2005 Sep; 2(3): 285–299.* doi: 10.1093/ecam/neh107; PMCID: PMC1193547. https://www.ncbi.nlm.nih.gov/pmc/articles/PMC1193547/

[66] Wang L, Hou Y (2011). Determination of trace elements in anti-influenza virus

mushrooms. *Biol Trace Elem Res. 2011 Dec;143(3):1799-807.* doi: 10.1007/s12011-011-8986-0; PMID: 21301988. https://www.ncbi.nlm.nih.gov/pubmed/21301988

[67] Alena G. Guggenheim, ND, Kirsten M. Wright, BS, and Heather L. Zwickey, PhD (2014). Immune Modulation From Five Major Mushrooms: Application to Integrative Oncology. *Integr Med (Encinitas). 2014 Feb; 13(1): 32–44.* PMCID: PMC4684115. https://www.ncbi.nlm.nih.gov/pmc/articles/PMC4684115/

[68] Homeopathy use around the world. Retrieved May 23, 2017 from Homeopathy Research Institute. https://www.hri-research.org/resources/homeopathy-the-debate/essentialevidence/use-of-homeopathy-across-the-world/

[69] Julian Winston. Treatment of Epidemics with Homeopathy - A History. Retrieved May 27, 2017 from National Centre for Homeopathy http://www.homeopathycenter.org/treatment-epidemics-homeopathy-history

[70] Elmira Akbari, Zatollah Asemi, Reza Daneshvar Kakhaki, Fereshteh Bahmani, Ebrahim Kouchaki, Omid Reza Tamtaji, Gholam Ali Hamidi, and Mahmoud Salami (2016). Effect of Probiotic Supplementation on Cognitive Function and Metabolic Status in Alzheimer's Disease: A Randomized, Double-Blind and Controlled Trial. *Front Aging Neurosci. 2016; 8: 256.* doi: 10.3389/fnagi.2016.00256; PMCID: PMC5105117. https://www.ncbi.nlm.nih.gov/pmc/articles/PMC5105117/

[71] Hsin-Jung Wu and Eric Wu (2012). The role of gut microbiota in immune homeostasis and autoimmunity. *Gut Microbes. 2012 Jan 1; 3(1): 4–14.* doi: 10.4161/gmic.19320; PMCID: PMC3337124. https://www.ncbi.nlm.nih.gov/pmc/articles/PMC3337124/

[72] Purchiaroni F, Tortora A, Gabrielli M, Bertucci F, Gigante G, Ianiro G, Ojetti V, Scarpellini E, Gasbarrini A. (2013). The role of intestinal microbiota and the immune system. *Eur Rev Med Pharmacol Sci. 2013 Feb;17(3):323-33.* PMID: 23426535. https://www.ncbi.nlm.nih.gov/pubmed/23426535

[73] Hyun Ho Choi and Young-Seok Cho (2016). Fecal Microbiota Transplantation: Current Applications, Effectiveness, and Future Perspectives. *Clin Endosc. 2016 May; 49(3): 257–265.* doi: 10.5946/ce.2015.117; PMCID: PMC4895930. https://www.ncbi.nlm.nih.gov/pmc/articles/PMC4895930/

[74] Jessica Wilks, Helen Beilinson, and Tatyana V. Golovkina (2013). Dual role of commensal bacteria in viral infections. *Immunol Rev. 2013 Sep; 255(1): 10.1111/imr.12097.* doi: 10.1111/imr.12097; PMCID: PMC3838194. https://www.ncbi.nlm.nih.gov/pmc/articles/PMC3838194/

[75] Takeshi Ichinohe, Iris K. Pang, Yosuke Kumamoto,a David R. Peaper,c John H. Ho,corresponding authora Thomas S. Murray,c,d and Akiko Iwasaki (2011). Microbiota regulates immune defense against respiratory tract influenza A virus infection. *Proc Natl Acad Sci U S A. 2011 Mar 29; 108(13): 5354–5359.* doi: 10.1073/pnas.1019378108; PMCID: PMC3069176.

https://www.ncbi.nlm.nih.gov/pmc/articles/PMC3069176/

[76] ibid

[77] Jian Wang, Fengqi Li, Rui Sun, Xiang Gao, Haiming Wei, Lan-Juan Li, and Zhigang Tiana (2013). Bacterial colonization dampens influenza-mediated acute lung injury via induction of M2 alveolar macrophages. *Nat Commun. 2013 Jul 3; 4: 2106.* doi: 10.1038/ncomms3106; PMCID: PMC3715851. https://www.ncbi.nlm.nih.gov/pmc/articles/PMC3715851/

[78] Ying Taur, MD, MPH and Eric G. Pamer, MD (2015). The Intestinal Microbiota and Susceptibility to Infection in Immunocompromised Patients. *Curr Opin Infect Dis. 2013 Aug; 26(4): 332–337.*doi: 10.1097/QCO.0b013e3283630dd3; PMCID: PMC4485384. https://www.ncbi.nlm.nih.gov/pmc/articles/PMC4485384/

[79] En-Jin Kang, Soo Young Kim,corresponding author In-Hong Hwang, and Yun-Jeong Ji (2013). The Effect of Probiotics on Prevention of Common Cold: A Meta-Analysis of Randomized Controlled Trial Studies. *Korean J Fam Med. 2013 Jan; 34(1): 2–10.* doi: 10.4082/kjfm.2013.34.1.2; PMCID: PMC3560336. https://www.ncbi.nlm.nih.gov/pmc/articles/PMC3560336/

[80] Joanne Slavin (2013). Fiber and Prebiotics: Mechanisms and Health Benefits. *Nutrients. 2013 Apr; 5(4): 1417–1435.* doi: 10.3390/nu5041417; PMCID: PMC3705355. https://www.ncbi.nlm.nih.gov/pmc/articles/PMC3705355/

[81] Shehata AA, Schrödl W, Aldin AA, Hafez HM, Krüger M.(2013). The effect of glyphosate on potential pathogens and beneficial members of poultry microbiota in vitro. *Curr Microbiol. 2013 Apr;66(4):350-8.* doi: 10.1007/s00284-012-0277-2; PMID: 23224412. https://www.ncbi.nlm.nih.gov/pubmed/23224412

[82] Nagai T, Makino S, Ikegami S, Itoh H, Yamada H. (2011). Effects of oral administration of yogurt fermented with Lactobacillus delbrueckii ssp. bulgaricus OLL1073R-1 and its exopolysaccharides against influenza virus infection in mice. *Int Immunopharmacol. 2011 Dec;11(12):2246-50.* doi: 10.1016/j.intimp.2011.09.012; PMID: 21986509. https://www.ncbi.nlm.nih.gov/pubmed/21986509

[83] N Waki, M Matsumoto, Y Fukui, and H Suganuma (2014). Effects of probiotic Lactobacillus brevis KB290 on incidence of influenza infection among schoolchildren: an open-label pilot study. *Lett Appl Microbiol. 2014 Dec; 59(6): 565–571.* doi: 10.1111/lam.12340; PMCID: PMC4285317. https://www.ncbi.nlm.nih.gov/pmc/articles/PMC4285317/

[84] Min-Kyung Park, Vu NGO, Young-Man Kwon, Young-Tae Lee, Sieun Yoo, Young-Hee Cho, Sung-Moon Hong, Hye Suk Hwang, Eun-Ju Ko, Yu-Jin Jung, Dae-Won Moon, Eun-Ji Jeong, Min-Chul Kim, Yu-Na Lee, Ji-Hun Jang, Joon-Suk Oh, Cheol-Hyun Kim, and Sang-Moo Kang (2013). Lactobacillus plantarum DK119 as a Probiotic Confers Protection against Influenza Virus by Modulating Innate

Immunity. *PLoS One. 2013; 8(10): e75368.* doi:
10.1371/journal.pone.0075368; PMCID: PMC3790790.
https://www.ncbi.nlm.nih.gov/pmc/articles/PMC3790790/

85 Funk C., Kennedy B., Public views about Americans' eating habits (2016).
http://www.pewinternet.org/2016/12/01/public-views-about-americans-eating-habits/

86 Rogers MAM, Aronoff DM (2016). The influence of non-steroidal anti-inflammatory drugs on the gut microbiome. *Clin Microbiol Infect. 2016 Feb;22(2):178.e1-178.e9.* doi: 10.1016/j.cmi.2015.10.003; PMID: 26482265.
https://www.ncbi.nlm.nih.gov/pubmed/26482265

87 ibid

88 Measuring Outpatient Antibiotic Prescribing . Retrieved May 14, 2017 from Centers for Disease Control and Prevention. https://www.cdc.gov/antibiotic-use/community/programs-measurement/measuring-antibiotic-prescribing.html

89 Cheryl Hogue (2017). California to list glyphosate as a carcinogen. *Chem Eng News Volume 95 Issue 27 | p. 14.*
https://cen.acs.org/articles/95/i27/California-list-glyphosate-carcinogen.html

90 ibid

91 Channa Jayasumana, Sarath Gunatilake, and Priyantha Senanayake (2014). Glyphosate, Hard Water and Nephrotoxic Metals: Are They the Culprits Behind the Epidemic of Chronic Kidney Disease of Unknown Etiology in Sri Lanka? *Int J Environ Res Public Health. 2014 Feb; 11(2): 2125–2147.* doi: 10.3390/ijerph110202125; PMCID: PMC3945589.
https://www.ncbi.nlm.nih.gov/pmc/articles/PMC3945589/

92 Freya Kamel and Jane A. Hoppin (2004). Association of Pesticide Exposure with Neurologic Dysfunction and Disease. *Environ Health Perspect. 2004 Jun; 112(9): 950–958.* doi: 10.1289/ehp.7135; PMCID: PMC1247187.
https://www.ncbi.nlm.nih.gov/pmc/articles/PMC1247187/

93 Anthony Samsel and Stephanie Seneff (2013). Glyphosate, pathways to modern diseases II: Celiac sprue and gluten intolerance. *Interdiscip Toxicol. 2013 Dec; 6(4): 159–184.* doi: 10.2478/intox-2013-0026; PMCID: PMC3945755.
https://www.ncbi.nlm.nih.gov/pmc/articles/PMC3945755/

94 How Does Chlorine in Water Affect my Health? Retrieved June 11, 2017 from Global Healing Centre http://www.bioray.com/content/Chlorine.pdf

95 Fluoride Found To Cause Cancer, Damage Thyroid, And Destroy The Immune System. Retrieved June 20, 2017 from The Science of Eating.
http://thescienceofeating.com/2015/11/09/fluoride-found-to-cause-cancer-damage-thyroid-and-destroy-the-immune-system-heres-what-you-need-to-know/

96 Fluoridation status of some countries. Retrieved June 20, 2017 from

Fluoridation.com http://www.fluoridation.com/c-country.htm

[97] Lee GI, Saravia J, You D, Shrestha B, Jaligama S, Hebert VY, Dugas TR, Cormier SA (2014). Exposure to combustion generated environmentally persistent free radicals enhances severity of influenza virus infection. *Part Fibre Toxicol. 2014 Oct 30;11:57.* doi: 10.1186/s12989-014-0057-1; PMID: 25358535. https://www.ncbi.nlm.nih.gov/pubmed/25358535

[98] Closa D, Folch-Puy E.(2004). Oxygen free radicals and the systemic inflammatory response. *IUBMB Life. 2004 Apr;56(4):185-91.* doi: 10.1080/15216540410001701642; PMID: 15230345. https://www.ncbi.nlm.nih.gov/pubmed/15230345

[99] Total Cholesterol Levels Vs Mortality Data From 164 Countries. Retrieved Sept 5, 2017 from https://renegadewellness.files.wordpress.com/2011/02/cholesterol-mortality-chart.pdf

[100] RR Elmehdawi (2008). Hypolipidemia: A Word of Caution. *Libyan J Med. 2008; 3(2): 84–90.* doi: 10.4176/071221; PMID: PMC3074286. https://www.ncbi.nlm.nih.gov/pmc/articles/PMC3074286/

[101] Hidesuke Kaji (2013). High-Density Lipoproteins and the Immune System. *J Lipids. 2013; 2013: 684903.* doi: 10.1155/2013/684903; PMID: PMC3572698. https://www.ncbi.nlm.nih.gov/pmc/articles/PMC3572698/

[102] Alexandra V. Yamshchikov, MD, Nirali S. Desai, MD, Henry M. Blumberg, MD, Thomas R. Ziegler, MD, and Vin Tangpricha, MD, PhD (2010). Vitamin D For Treatment And Prevention Of Infectious Diseases: A Systematic Review Of Randomized Controlled Trials. *Endocr Pract. 2009 Jul–Aug; 15(5): 438–449.*doi: 10.4158/EP09101.ORR; PMCID: PMC2855046. https://www.ncbi.nlm.nih.gov/pmc/articles/PMC2855046/

[103] Martin A. Kriegel, MD, PhD, JoAnn E. Manson, MD, DrPH, and Karen H. Costenbader, MD, MPH (2011). Does Vitamin D Affect Risk of Developing Autoimmune Disease?: A Systematic Review. *Semin Arthritis Rheum. 2011 Jun; 40(6): 512–531.e8.* doi: 10.1016/j.semarthrit.2010.07.009; PMCID: PMC3098920. https://www.ncbi.nlm.nih.gov/pmc/articles/PMC3098920/

[104] Cedric F. Garland, DrPH, Frank C. Garland, PhD, Edward D. Gorham, PhD, MPH, Martin Lipkin, MD, Harold Newmark, ScD, Sharif B. Mohr, MPH, and Michael F. Holick, MD, PhD (2006). The Role of Vitamin D in Cancer Prevention. *Am J Public Health. 2006 February; 96(2): 252–261.* doi: 10.2105/AJPH.2004.045260; PMCID: PMC1470481. https://www.ncbi.nlm.nih.gov/pmc/articles/PMC1470481/

48186362R00083

Made in the USA
Columbia, SC
06 January 2019